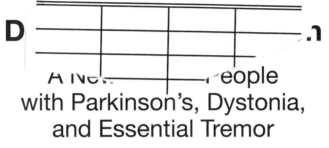

D _____ ᴉ

A Neᵥ _____ ᵣeople
with Parkinson's, Dystonia,
and Essential Tremor

Kelvin L. Chou, MD
Susan Grube, RN, MSN
Parag G. Patil, MD, PhD

Visit our website at www.demoshealth.com

ISBN: 978-1-936303-11-3
e-book ISBN: 978-1-617050-63-3

Acquisitions Editor: Noreen Henson
Compositor: Manila Typesetting Company

Library of Congress Cataloging-in-Publication Data

Chou, Kelvin L.
  Deep brain stimulation : a new life for people with Parkinson's, dystonia and essential tremor / Kelvin L. Chou, Susan Grube, Parag G. Patil.
     p. cm.
  Includes bibliographical references and index.
  ISBN 978-1-936303-11-3 (pbk.)
  1. Brain stimulation. 2. Movement disorders--Treatment. I. Grube, Susan. II. Patil, Parag G. III. Title.
  RC350.B72C48 2012
  616.8--dc23
                                                            2011039580

Special discounts on bulk quantities of Demos Health books are available to corporations, professional associations, pharmaceutical companies, health care organizations, and other qualifying groups. For details, please contact:

Special Sales Department
Demos Medical Publishing, LLC
11 West 42nd Street, 15th Floor
New York, NY 10036
Phone: 800-532-8663 or 212-683-0072
Fax: 212-941-7842
E-mail: rsantana@demosmedpub.com

Printed in the United States of America by Bang Printing.
11 12 13 14 / 5 4 3 2 1

Table of Contents

Foreword

If you're thinking about having DBS for a neurological problem, read this book. It explains exactly how the process of selecting patients is made, what steps are necessary before surgery, what happens during surgery, and what happens after surgery. Each step of the lengthy process is discussed in detail. Pictures and photos illustrate much of the process. Time estimates are even provided so you will understand why the surgery takes so long; what placement of "the frame" means; and what to expect on completing the surgery. These authors discuss financial aspects of the surgery and how the results of surgery may affect the family and social support system. It is an all-inclusive discussion that should help quell anxieties while you're waiting or deciding. There is a glossary to help you understand any technical terms you are bound to come across on the internet or in any discussion.

DBS is, at least for most of us, still something of a "science fiction" type approach to treating an illness although it's been an FDA approved treatment for many years, paid for by all medical insurers. These authors are, however, very much grounded in reality. They have lots of experience and have been through thick and thin with many, many patients (including my own), experiencing the wonderful joy of the great successes but they've also been there for the patients with the side effects or the disappointing responses. While there is little so rewarding for a health professional as when a patient describes the surgery as "my second birthday," there is also little so disappointing as a treatment failure.

These authors present an accurate and balanced picture of DBS and make it clear that it always represents the choice made by weighing the risks and potential side effects. This is not curative surgery. It is one treatment approach, like a medication. Where the balance point is located for making the decision differs for each individual, as this book makes very clear.

A frequent radio advertisement for a clothing store notes that, "An educated consumer is our best customer." That certainly applies to DBS surgery. Take the time to learn all you can. This book will help.

Joseph H. Friedman, MD
Director, Movement Disorders Program
Butler Hospital
Department of Neurology
Alpert Medical School of Brown University
Providence, Rhode Island

ONE

A Little History on Deep Brain Stimulation

DEEP BRAIN STIMULATION THERAPY

A deep brain stimulator (DBS) device is similar to a pacemaker for the heart, but instead of having electrodes (or electrical wires) implanted in the heart, the electrodes are placed into the brain. The electrodes carry electrical signals to specific brain locations. These electrical signals, like a heart pacemaker, cause the brain cells around the DBS electrode to change their activity. By changing the activity of brain cells, DBS can help the symptoms of many neurological disorders, depending on where the electrodes are placed.

Diseases treated with DBS include Parkinson's disease, essential tremor (ET), dystonia, and a few other neurological and psychiatric disorders. Parkinson's disease, essential tremor, and dystonia are examples of movement disorders. Movement disorders are neurological diseases that affect the ability to produce and control movements of the body. In individuals with these conditions, the firing patterns of nerve cells within certain parts of the brain become abnormal. These abnormal patterns spread through the electrical circuits of the brain to other areas such as the brain areas connected to the spinal cord that guide movement, the brain areas that steady the limbs and smooth movement, or the brain areas that help to start and stop movements. The abnormal activity in these brain circuits creates the symptoms of the disease condition, such as tremor in Parkinson's disease and essential tremor or the abnormal muscle contractions in dystonia.

UNDERSTANDING THE MOTOR SYSTEM OF THE BRAIN

The way we move requires a lot of processes to occur in the brain in a coordinated way. Today, we know that there are two systems (or types of circuits) in the brain that control movement.

The "pyramidal system" is one of these motor circuits. It is composed of cells that directly control the motor neurons (or nerve cells) of the spinal cord. The principal area of the brain containing these cells is the primary motor cortex, which is located on the surface of the brain, just above the ear. Cells in this region extend portions of themselves (known as processes) down through a bundle of nerves called the internal capsule, through the brainstem (the connection between the brain and the spinal cord), and eventually to the spinal cord. The pyramidal system itself is named after the pyramid shape of these processes in the brainstem.

The "extrapyramidal system" is the second motor system of the brain. It is composed of the circuits of the brain whose fibers do not travel through the pyramids. The extrapyramidal circuits shape movement by influencing our reflexes, coordination, and posture. These circuits also break down our complex movements into sequences of simple ones.

The pyramidal system is largely located in the surface portion of the brain: the cerebral cortex. The extrapyramidal system is located deep within the brain, in structures such as the basal ganglia, brainstem, and cerebellum.

When we move as a result of a desire or goal, the movements are voluntary. When we move without such a desire, such as when we experience a tremor, the movements become involuntary. DBS systems are placed into extrapyramidal motor system circuits to control and reduce involuntary movements.

HISTORICAL UNDERSTANDING OF THE DISEASES TREATED WITH DBS

Parkinson's Disease

Although the terms "Parkinson's disease," "essential tremor," and "dystonia" were first used a century or more ago, these diseases have been known and treated for centuries. The disease now known as Parkinson's disease was described and treated as early as 5000 BC by ancient civilizations in India that termed the disease "Kampavata." Kampavata was treated with a tropical plant containing natural quantities of levodopa, one of the best medications for the treatment of Parkinson's disease today. James Parkinson (1755–1824) was an English physician who first described the symptoms of the disease that now bears his name in a manuscript called "An Essay on the Shaking

Palsy" in 1817. His description of the symptoms of Parkinson's disease was remarkably accurate, especially because it was based on just six people, three of whom he did not even see in his practice, but observed on his daily walks. In the Western world, the first treatment of Parkinson's disease was the use of belladonna drops by Jean-Martin Charcot (1825–1883) to treat the excessive salivation that occurred in some individuals. It was Charcot who recommended that the disease be named after James Parkinson.

Essential Tremor

Essential tremor has also been known since the ancient times. The Greek physician Galen (130–200 AD) wrote of an action tremor condition in his essay "De Tremore" between 169 and 180 AD. Other ancient accounts of essential tremor occur in the medical publications of Israel and India. Pietro Burresi was the first to use the term "tremore semplice essenziale," or essential tremor, in 1874 to describe an 18-year-old man with a severe tremor of the arms when moving them. Dr. Charles Dana (1852–1935), a New York neurologist, was one of the first to extensively study essential tremor, publishing a study of several large families in 1887. Essential tremor has been treated with a class of medications known as beta-blockers since the 1960s [of which propranolol (Inderal) is the most commonly used] and with anticonvulsant medications such as mysoline (Primidone) since the late 1970s.

Dystonia

Dystonia has been also recognized for centuries. In fact, individuals with dystonia are often depicted in ancient works of art. In modern times, Hermann Oppenheim (1858–1919) applied the term "dystonia musculorum deformans" to four children with a progressive, generalized dystonia in 1911 and was the first to recognize dystonia as a movement disorder. Before Oppenheim, many physicians mistakenly believed dystonia to be a purely psychiatric disorder. Dystonia has been treated with anticholinergic medications such as trihexylphenidyl (Artane) since the 1950s and with muscle relaxants such as baclofen (Lioresal) since the 1960s.

EARLY BRAIN SURGERIES FOR MOVEMENT DISORDERS

The earliest surgeries for movement disorders were directed at the muscles producing the movements themselves rather than the brain.

For example, surgery for dystonia was first performed in 1641 by the German surgeon Isaac Minnius and involved cutting the muscles in the neck that were involved in cervical (neck) dystonia (also known as torticollis).

During the 19th century, understanding of the regions of the brain involved in movement helped motivate surgeons to address movement disorders through operations on the brain. Gustav Fritsch (1838–1927) and Eduard Hitzig (1838–1907) reported experiments that helped to localize motor function in the cerebral cortex (the surface of the brain) in 1870. The earliest surgeries for movement disorders therefore involved removing these surface areas of the brain. These surgeries eliminated abnormal movements, but unfortunately, it caused weakness. Victor Horsley (1857–1916), a British surgeon, was the first to describe a procedure in which the primary motor cortex was removed to treat tremor. A. Earl Walker (1907–1995), an American, later described a less invasive procedure in which the nerve fibers of primary motor cortex cells, connecting the brain to the spinal cord, were partially cut to produce both weakness and relief of tremor. This procedure, called pedunculectomy, remained popular until the 1950s.

In the 1920s and 1930s, the role of the extrapyramidal system in movement disorders became more widely appreciated. Otfrid Foerster (1873–1941), Cecile Vogt (1875–1962), and Oskar Vogt (1870–1959) demonstrated that changes in the deeper structures in the brain were fundamentally involved in Parkinson's disease and other movement disorders. Rolf Hassler (1914–1984) observed that Parkinson's disease was associated with the loss of pigmented nerve cells in the substantia nigra. We now know that these pigmented nerve cells are dopamine-producing cells, and that the loss of these cells results in loss of dopamine in the brain, causing symptoms of Parkinson's disease. Building on these findings, and those of others, Hugo Spatz (1888–1969) defined the extrapyramidal regions of the brain and proposed that movement disorders arose within this system.

Based on these findings, neurosurgeons developed surgeries directed toward the extrapyramidal motor system.

In 1942, Russell Meyers (1904–1999) first reported the effects of surgery on the basal ganglia (a major group of structures within the extrapyramidal system) for Parkinson's disease. He removed the head and anterior segment of the caudate nucleus, one of the structures of the basal ganglia, and found that tremor and rigidity improved without the creation of weakness. Later surgeons improved on his technique, introducing the idea of using intense heat or cold to create a permanent lesion in the brain.

Some of the progress in brain surgery for movement disorders came by accident. Irving Cooper (1922–1985) was performing Walker's pedunculectomy operation for tremor in 1952, and during the operation, noted bleeding forced him to stop. To his surprise, the tremor was eliminated, although the actual goal of the surgery was not achieved. Cooper knew which blood vessel had been injured in the surgery and reasoned that the area of the brain that was fed by the blood vessel must have been injured. He reasoned that intentionally injuring this area might improve tremor. This finding directed attention toward the pallidum, another structure in the basal ganglia, as a target for movement disorder surgery.

Once doctors treating movement disorders realized that lesions (or injuries) of specific structures deep within the brain could treat individuals safely and effectively, surgery for movement disorders began in earnest. To allow more precise targeting of structures deep within the brain, clinical neuroscientists and neurosurgeons developed methods of image-directed surgery. In 1947, Ernest Spiegel and Henry Wycis introduced the first frame-based human surgeries. The stereotactic frame is a metal device that is attached to the skull and allows precise targeting of structures within the skull by associating a coordinate system with structures within the skull. Lars Leksell (1907–1986), a Swedish neurosurgeon, introduced a more simply designed frame in 1949. Versions of these frames are used to this day.

Frame-based stereotactic surgery was performed extensively in the 1950s and 1960s. By utilizing a frame, internal brain structures could be reproducibly targeted. The two primary targets of surgery were the pallidum and the thalamus, and these structures were lesioned by burning or freezing the brain tissue in that area. Hirotaro Narabayashi (1922-2001) performed the first human stereotactic pallidotomy (destruction of cells in the pallidum) in 1951. Rolf Hassler described stereotactic lesioning of the ventral intermediate (VIM) nucleus of the thalamus for parkinsonian tremor in 1954.

In 1968, George Cotzias (1918–1977) discovered and developed a way to give levodopa to people living with Parkinson's in large-enough doses to treat the symptoms with minimal side effects. Levodopa was (and still remains) an effective therapy for the symptoms of Parkinson's disease. Because of this, the risks of surgery exceeded the risks of medical therapy, and the number of surgeries for Parkinson's disease dropped dramatically.

ELECTRICAL THERAPIES IN THE BRAIN

Today, we take it for granted that the brain is an electrical organ and that the cells of the brain communicate with each other through chemical and electrical signals. However, the role of electricity in the body was not always known. Luigi Galvani (1737–1798) reported that electrical stimulation could produce contractions in frog muscles in 1791. His nephew, Giovani Aldini (1762–1834), was the first to demonstrate the therapeutic role of electricity in the human nervous system, in 1801, using electricity to treat a person with depression.

During the 19th century, understanding of the electrical characteristics of the brain increased significantly. Fritsch and Hitzig utilized electrical stimulation to study the motor function in the brain in 1870. These findings were extended in the work of David Ferrier (1842–1928) and Robert Bartholow (1831–1904).

Although electrical stimulation in the form of individual shocks was utilized to treat depression in the 18th century, the technology to produce reliable ongoing stimulation was not available until the 20th century. In 1948, J. Lawrence Pool (1906–2004) was the first neurosurgeon to utilize deep brain stimulation in a person living with Parkinson's disease. This individual, who suffered from appetite loss and depression associated with Parkinson's disease, was treated for eight weeks with stimulation of the caudate, yet another basal ganglia structure. At the time, brain stimulation was primarily used to predict the outcomes of stereotactic lesions in the brain, particularly for the treatment of pain. Less frequently, stimulation and lesions to the thalamus, pallidum, and cerebellum were performed for the treatment of tremor. This practice continued until the 1960s, when the demand for movement disorder surgery was reduced after the introduction of levodopa.

DEEP BRAIN STIMULATION IN THE MODERN ERA

Yoshio Hosobuchi first performed chronic deep brain stimulation using implanted electrodes for the treatment of pain in 1973. The technology was adapted from the heart pacemaker, which had been introduced in 1958. In the early years, DBS was applied to regions of the brain controlling pain as well the cerebellum to treat spasticity and tremor.

A French neurosurgeon, Alim Louis Benabid, noticed in 1987 that chronic stimulation in the thalamus resulted in the disappearance of tremor. Chronic stimulation was used to confirm the precise location in the brain that was going to be lesioned. Instead of making a lesion in this patient, he decided to implant a deep brain stimulator at that location instead. In 1993, he reported the impressive results of long-term deep brain stimulation on tremor. The long-term results of pallidal stimulation for Parkinson's disease were reported in 2002. With these final steps forward, the field of DBS was born.

TWO

How Does DBS Work and What Can It Do for Me?

As mentioned in the last chapter, deep brain stimulation (DBS) therapy involves the placement of electrical wires in certain areas of the brain. Through these wires, electrical stimulation is delivered to the brain and helps to improve the symptoms of certain conditions. Today, DBS is an established surgical treatment approved by the U.S. Food and Drug Administration (FDA) to control the symptoms of Parkinson's disease, essential tremor, and dystonia. For people with Parkinson's, DBS can reduce tremors and significantly improve slowness and stiffness. For people with essential tremor, DBS can make the tremors disappear, allowing them to eat and drink without spilling. For people with dystonia, DBS can relax the muscles, improve abnormal postures caused by muscle contractions, and improve quality of life. This therapy can be life-changing and allow people to do simple things they had been unable to do for years. To understand how DBS works, it helps to first know the parts of the DBS system that are placed in the body.

THE DBS SYSTEM

The deep brain stimulation system consists of three separate parts: the DBS lead, an extension wire, and the stimulator:

1. **Lead:** The DBS lead is the portion of the system that is located in the brain. The lead is about the size of a thin and extralong piece of spaghetti (1.2 mm × 40 cm or approximately 1/20 in. × 16 in.). It is a hollow tube that contains four individually insulated wires. The end of the lead is placed into a specific area in the brain and has four metal rings that come into contact with the brain. These rings are called "contacts." The contacts are 1.5 mm in length and are

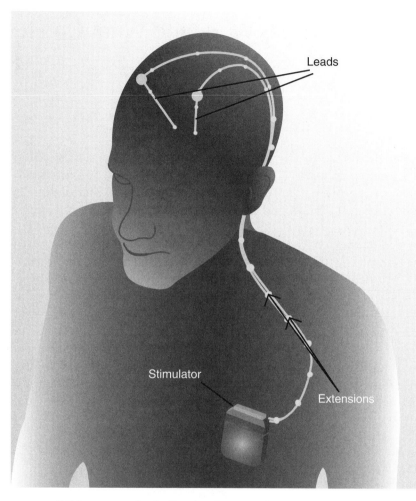

DBS system, including lead, extension, and stimulator

spaced 0.5–1.5 mm apart depending on the model. Electrical stimulation comes out of these contacts and delivers electrical energy to the area surrounding the contact.

2. **Extension:** A wire that carries the electrical stimulation from the stimulator to the lead. A connector fits the extension wire to the lead on one end and plugs into the stimulator on the other end with two prongs. The extension comes in a variety of sizes and is made of insulated wires wrapped in silicone rubber. This allows the extension lead to be flexible, strong, and waterproof.

3. **Stimulator:** A pacemaker-like device containing a battery that is the source of the electrical signals that eventually travel to the contacts in the DBS lead. This part may also be referred to as the "battery," the "pacemaker," or the "implantable pulse generator" (IPG). Depending on the model of the stimulator, the size and thickness may vary, but it is typically the thickness of half of a deck of playing cards and slightly shorter than a business card. The IPG battery and circuits are protected from the outside world by a metal casing. In addition, the IPG contains a connector that allows it to be attached to the rest of the DBS system.

This entire three-part system is implanted inside the body, under the skin, so there are no parts exposed to the air. The design of the DBS system has proven to be a highly durable one. Although damage to the DBS system does occur occasionally (such as a break in the wire or lead), the hardware is strong and flexible enough that most individuals can lead active lives, playing golf and doing other physical activities, without worrying about damaging the system.

A lead may be placed on one side or both sides of the brain, depending on an individual's particular condition. When it is placed on one side of the brain, it is called *unilateral* stimulation, and when it is placed on both sides of the brain, it is called *bilateral* stimulation. One of the most important features of DBS is that it is programmable. This means that the characteristics of the electrical pulses can be set through a remote control that is outside of the body. The remote control can set the frequency (how many times per second) at which an electrical pulse occurs (usually 130–185 pulses per second), the width of the electrical pulse (usually 60 millionths of a second or microseconds), and the strength of the pulse (usually 1–4 V). The remote control can also set which contacts at the tip of the lead will deliver the electrical stimulation.

The only DBS system approved by the FDA for use at the time of this publication is made by Medtronic, Inc. They have several models. The oldest model is the Soletra, which connects one lead to one extension and one stimulator. If an individual needs bilateral stimulation, two Soletras would be implanted, one on each side. The Kinetra allows two leads and extensions to be plugged into one stimulator. Most recent on the market are the Activa PC and Activa RC. The Activa PC is similar to the Kinetra but has slightly more features. The Activa RC is a rechargeable battery. The choice of the model is often decided by the surgical team based on familiarity and cost (what insurance will reimburse). St. Jude Medical also produces a DBS system that has undergone clinical trials and is approved for use in Europe. However, it has not yet been approved in the U.S. by the FDA as of this printing. If it does receive approval, there will be more choice and competition on the market, which will likely be good for everyone overall.

THE SKINNY ON HOW DBS WORKS AND WHAT IT CAN DO

How exactly does DBS work in the brain to make all this happen? That question is currently being debated by scientists all over the world. The short answer to this question is: we do not know exactly. However, there are different explanations for how DBS works that depend on the condition being treated. In this section, we describe how DBS works and what DBS can do for people living with Parkinson's disease, essential tremor, and dystonia.

For Parkinson's Disease

To understand how DBS works for Parkinson's disease, you must first understand the symptoms of the disease and what causes them in the brain. Parkinson's disease is a slowly progressive neurological disorder that affects the movement of the body. It typically affects people as they get older, with an average age of onset in the mid-60s. The three main motor symptoms of Parkinson's disease are shaking (or *tremor*), slowness of movement (also called *bradykinesia*), and stiffness (or *rigidity*). The *tremor* in Parkinson's disease is most noticeable in the arms or legs when they are at rest and tends to improve when the arms or legs are in use. For example, a hand tremor in Parkinson's disease can be noticeable when the hand is resting on the lap, but will often disappear when a person uses that hand to eat or write. *Bradykinesia* refers to a slowness of movement, although people may describe this slowness as "weakness" or "incoordination." Bradykinesia can cause slowness and difficulty with tasks such as buttoning clothes, tying shoelaces, typing, or lifting coins from a pocket or purse. It may also cause someone with Parkinson's to drag the legs or take shorter steps when walking. *Rigidity* often causes stiffened movement of the arms, legs, or body and may cause pain or soreness in these areas.

What happens in the brain to cause these motor symptoms of Parkinson's disease? We talked about the extrapyramidal system in Chapter 1, which is one of the motor systems in the brain that coordinates movement. A part of the extrapyramidal system, the basal ganglia, is involved in Parkinson's disease. Normally, certain nerve cells (or neurons) in the basal ganglia make a chemical called dopamine. In people with Parkinson's disease, these nerve cells slowly stop working or die, so the brain loses its ability to produce dopamine. The loss of dopamine causes the shaking, slowed movements, and stiffness of Parkinson's. It is estimated that anywhere between 50% and 75% of your dopamine-producing cells are already gone when you first start noticing the motor symptoms of Parkinson's, but it is not yet clear how or why these cells stop working correctly.

When dopamine is lost in the brain, the normal electrical activity in the basal ganglia becomes different. This affects the messages that your brain sends down to your body. When deep brain stimulation was first discovered, it was thought that maybe it silenced the nerve cells around the electrode, similar to what happened with lesioning procedures. By silencing the electrical activity that was abnormal, it allowed the normal messages from your brain to your body to go through. Although this is an attractive explanation, we now know that the way DBS works in Parkinson's is not by silencing the cells. Instead, the abnormal electrical activity caused by loss of dopamine seems to be replaced with a different electrical signal that allows the messages to get through better. However, this different signal is still different from the normal electrical activity of the brain.

There is a famous "I Love Lucy" scene where Lucy and her friend Ethel try to find some work, while their husbands stay at home to see if they can run a household. Lucy and Ethel eventually get hired to work in the wrapping department of a candy shop. They sit down in front of a conveyor belt and are instructed that each piece of candy that comes down the belt must be wrapped before it gets packed into a box. At first, the conveyor belt moves slowly, and Lucy and Ethel have no problem performing their job. However, the candy starts coming out faster and faster, and Lucy and Ethel cannot keep up. When their supervisor comes out, they end up eating some of the candy or stuffing some of the candy in their hats and shirts to disguise how hopeless they are at their job. Think of the candy factory as the brain and Lucy and Ethel as the basal ganglia. Lucy and Ethel cannot keep up with the signals (the candy) coming from the brain, and as a result, the signals get messed up (gets eaten or stuffed in hats). In a normal brain (or candy shop), two workers should be able to keep up with the flow of signals (chocolate) coming from the brain (conveyor belt). What deep brain stimulation does is add two more workers to the candy shop (changes the electrical signal) rather than fix the original workers (restoring normal signal). Now four workers are better able to handle the flow of candy coming down the conveyor belt, but it is still not the same as what a normal candy shop should be able to do.

When thinking about what deep brain stimulation can do for you if you have Parkinson's, it is first important to know what the medications can do. The medications used to treat Parkinson's disease concentrate on replacing the dopamine that is lost. As mentioned in Chapter 1, one of the best medications for the motor symptoms of Parkinson's is called levodopa. It is often paired with carbidopa in the U.S. and benserazide in other countries. Carbidopa and benserazide prevent levodopa from being broken down before it gets to the brain. In the U.S., the combination of carbidopa and levodopa is marketed as Sinemet. Levodopa gets absorbed in the intestine, travels to the brain, and gets converted by the brain's own cells to dopamine. Other medications for Parkinson's disease are aimed at enhancing the dopamine system in the brain. For example, there are medications that prevent the breakdown of dopamine in the brain and allow it to last longer [catechol-O-methyl-transferase (COMT) or monoamine oxidase B (MAO-B) inhibitors]. Dopamine agonists are medications that resemble dopamine and act on the dopamine receptors in the brain. Most of these medications help the motor symptoms of Parkinson's, but levodopa is the best of them all. People living with Parkinson's disease who take levodopa can feel normal, and the tremors, slowness, and stiffness can disappear when on the medication. Early in the disease, levodopa can last many, many hours. Unfortunately, as time goes on, the levodopa effect does not last as long. People who once took levodopa every 8 hours may find themselves taking it every 6 hours, then every 4 hours, then every 3 hours, etc. When levodopa works, individuals feel good and have good motor function (this is called "on" time). However, when the medication wears off, people feel slow, stiff, and generally worse (this is called "off" time).

People who are on levodopa may also notice *dyskinesias*. Dyskinesias are abnormal, involuntary movements that in their mildest form make one resemble a very fidgety person, but, when severe, can make someone look like he or she is constantly in motion. If you have seen Michael J. Fox in an interview recently, you may be able to see what dyskinesias look like.

Deep brain stimulation was approved for Parkinson's disease by the FDA in 2002. It helps to relieve these motor symptoms and has a similar effect to levodopa—it reduces stiffness and improves the ability to move. DBS may also reduce the severity of tremor. The one main difference between DBS and levodopa, however, is that the former, over time, relieves *dyskinesias*, whereas the latter, over time, causes *dyskinesias*. Furthermore, because electrical stimulation is constantly delivered to the brain, 24 hours a day, 7 days a week, people experience an increase in their "on" time (when the motor function is good). Medication "off" times (when the motor function is poor) with DBS are typically shorter and milder than before surgery. It is important to remember that DBS will not make you better than your best "on" time, but it can help you to experience your best "on" time for a longer portion of the day. Most people continue their Parkinson's medications after surgery, but the amount or frequency of the medication may decrease. This is an additional benefit of surgery, but it is not the goal.

DBS for Parkinson's Disease

A 64-year-old woman developed a right-hand rest tremor 17 years ago. The rest tremor was mild, and she did not require treatment for 5 years. The tremor then became more consistent and was accompanied by clumsiness in the right hand and generalized slowness. She was initially started on low doses of levodopa, which gave her complete control of her symptoms. She required higher doses of levodopa over the following years as her symptoms spread to the left side of her body. Other medications were added over the years, but despite all of her medications, she began to experience wearing-off symptoms and dyskinesias. In the few years prior to DBS, she had severe motor fluctuations. When the medications were working for her (about three-fourths of the day), she was able to move but had severe dyskinesias. When she was "off" medications (about one-fourth of the day), she reported being almost unable to move.

She underwent DBS surgery, where the electrodes were placed in the subthalamic nuclei on both sides of the brain. Six months after surgery, after her stimulator settings were optimized, she did not have any significant wearing off or dyskinesias. In addition, she was able to reduce her dopaminergic medications by about 90%. She felt that she had been "given her life back."

For Parkinson's disease, there are three different sites in the brain where the DBS electrodes can be placed: the ventralis intermedius (VIM) nucleus of the thalamus, the globus pallidus interna (GPi), or the subthalamic nucleus (STN). Most deep brain stimulation centers worldwide tend to place the electrodes in the STN for people living with Parkinson's mainly because of training and comfort. One recent large study comparing STN stimulation to GPi stimulation for Parkinson's disease demonstrated that they were similar in terms of improvement in motor symptoms. However, individuals were able to reduce their medications more with STN stimulation compared with GPi stimulation. Stimulating the thalamus in Parkinson's disease only helps

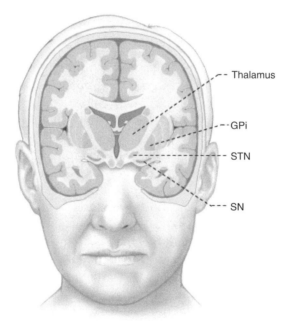

Sites for deep brain stimulation, thalamus, GPi, and STN
(SN stands for substantia nigra, the site in the brain where
dopamine nerve cells degenerate)
Source: Hubert H. Fernandez, Ramon L. Rodriguez, Frank M. Skidmore, and Michael S. Okun. *A Practical Guide to Movement Disorders.* New York: Demos Medical Publishing, 2007.

tremor, not bradykinesia or rigidity. Your DBS team may propose putting electrodes in the VIM thalamus only if tremor seems to be the biggest problem, and there is little in the way of bradykinesia or rigidity.

For Essential Tremor

What exactly is essential tremor (ET)? Essential tremor is a progressive neurological disorder that causes tremors, generally of both hands, but also the head and voice. It is often confused with Parkinson's disease, but the tremor in essential tremor is an action tremor, which means that the tremor occurs or is most noticeable when the limb is in use or moving. This is the opposite of the tremor seen in Parkinson's disease, which (as mentioned earlier in this chapter) is a tremor that is most noticeable when the limbs are relaxed or resting.

Because the hands and arms are typically the most commonly affected parts of the body in essential tremor, people who have this condition usually shake when they try to hold their arms out in front of them. Many tasks may be affected by essential tremor, and people may notice shaking when writing, typing, using a computer mouse, applying makeup, eating, or drinking from a glass of water. The shaking may get worse as the person is about to reach his or her goal. As an example, the shaking may be bad as a person drinks soup from a spoon, with the most severe tremor right as the spoon gets to the mouth.

We mentioned earlier that the tremors of essential tremor can also affect the head and the voice. Rarely are the legs affected. Essential tremor can start at any age, even as early as childhood, but typically worsens over time. It is also known as "benign tremor" or "benign essential tremor" because in many cases, it usually does not cause disability. However, in those people who have severe cases, "benign tremor" is probably not the best description. It is also clear that essential tremor runs in families. Because of this, it may also be called a "familial tremor" or "benign familial tremor" by some physicians. However, essential tremor may occur in someone without a clear family history.

Scientists do not know exactly what is going on in the brain to cause the symptoms of essential tremor, but it is thought that essential tremor results from improper regulation of activity in a cell group or circuit in the brain. There is increasing evidence from autopsied brains of those who were diagnosed with essential tremor that the brain abnormality involves the cerebellum or nerve fibers from the cerebellum. The cerebellum is a part of the brain in the back of the head that is involved in the control and coordination of movement. It sends fibers to the VIM thalamus, which is where the electrode tip is placed in individuals with essential tremor. High-frequency stimulation in the thalamus appears to override abnormal activity in this structure and replaces it with more regular firing. This, in turn, causes tremors in the hands to disappear.

According to the website of the International Essential Tremor Foundation (www.essentialtremor.org), up to 10 million Americans have essential tremor. However, many do not even seek medical attention because the tremors do not cause any limitations in lifestyle. For those with essential tremor who feel embarrassed or have difficulty performing basic tasks due to hand tremors, there are several medications available. Propranolol (Inderal) and mysoline (Primidone) are the main agents used. Other medications including topiramate (Topamax), clonazepam (Klonopin), and gabapentin (Neurontin) may also be used. Unfortunately, only about 60%–70% of people living with essential tremor will respond to medications.

The FDA approved DBS for the treatment of essential tremor in 1997. DBS significantly relieves tremor in this condition and improves quality of life. The DBS electrode is typically placed in the VIM thalamus on the side of the brain opposite the hand tremor. Thus, if the right hand has significant tremor, the DBS electrode is placed in the left thalamus. Unlike Parkinson's disease, where electrodes are placed on both sides of the brain, only one electrode is usually implanted for those living with essential tremor. This decreases surgical risks, as stimulation of both thalami may result in more unwanted side effects, especially with speech. Most of the studies looking at long-term outcomes of DBS for essential tremor have reported up to 90% improvement in hand tremor for up to 7 years. Head and voice tremor rarely improves with unilateral thalamic stimulation. To improve head and voice tremor, electrodes need to be placed on both sides of the brain, although, again, bilateral stimulation often causes problems with speech.

DBS for Essential Tremor

A 60-year-old woman first noticed tremor in her hands when she was 11 years old. The tremor was mild at first and involved only the hands, but as she got older, she developed a head tremor as well. The head tremor was never severe, but the hand tremors became more noticeable as she grew older. For the

5 years prior to DBS surgery, the hand tremors interfered with her eating and drinking. She was unable to drink from a regular cup without spilling and needed to use a straw while holding a cup with both hands. Eating food was difficult without spilling, and she felt too embarrassed to eat in public. She also had difficulty signing her name because of her tremors and reported difficulty brushing her teeth to the point where the tremor created an ulcer on the roof of her mouth.

She underwent deep brain stimulation surgery. Because she was right handed, a DBS electrode was placed in the left VIM thalamus to control her right-hand tremor. She reported crying the first time she was able to drink coffee from a mug using her right hand without spilling, and 3 months after surgery, she had no noticeable tremor in her right hand with the stimulator turned on.

For Dystonia

Dystonia is a neurological disorder where certain muscles start to involuntarily contract and spasm. This often results in twisting or repetitive movements and awkward or abnormal postures. Dystonias are often categorized into primary and secondary dystonias. Primary dystonias are either genetic (which means that they run in families) or without identifiable cause. In secondary dystonias, the dystonia results from something else. The causes of secondary dystonias are varied and include trauma, cerebral palsy, multiple sclerosis, tumor, stroke, and drugs. Even other neurologic disorders such as Parkinson's disease may cause dystonia. Dystonia can affect anyone: men, women, or children of any age or ethnicity. Approximately 300,000 people in North America are estimated to have dystonia.

The symptoms that a person with dystonia experiences depend on the part of the body that is affected. Dystonia may affect any part of the body. In childhood, dystonia usually starts in one limb such as the leg or arm but tends to spread and may involve the whole body (generalized dystonia). Dystonias that start in childhood often have a genetic cause. In adulthood, dystonias generally affect one body part such as the neck, face, or arm and tend to stay confined to that body part. Pain may also be a prominent part of some dystonias such as cervical (neck) dystonia. Because this condition causes progressive disability, many sufferers may have difficulty adapting, resulting in mood problems such as depression. Fortunately, dystonia generally does not affect thinking, memory, or intelligence.

Botulinum toxin is the preferred treatment for most dystonias that involve only one area of the body. It is given through injection into the affected muscle. The toxin then blocks the signal from the nerve to the muscle. Because the muscle never receives the signal to contract, it relaxes. Unfortunately, in people with generalized dystonia, too many different muscles are involved and too much botulinum toxin is needed to make it a practical treatment. For generalized dystonia, muscle relaxants, valium-like drugs, or a medication known as trihexyphenidyl (Artane) are typically prescribed.

The causes of primary dystonia are not yet known or understood. Secondary dystonias are those that have some identified cause. In primary dystonias of childhood onset, the cause is suspected to be due to a problem in the basal ganglia and is most often genetic. In primary dystonias of adult onset, environmental or task-related factors are suspected to trigger their development. What happens in the brain in dystonia is that the pattern of brain cell activity in the basal ganglia (the part of the brain that helps control movement) is changed. As in Parkinson's disease, DBS probably changes this abnormal pattern of activity and improves the dystonia.

DBS was approved by the FDA under a humanitarian device exemption for dystonia in 2003. What this means is that DBS was approved not because there was a lot of evidence that it is effective for dystonia, but because there is often minimal effect from other treatments. The brain target for dystonia is the GPi. For people who are unresponsive to medication, DBS therapy *may* significantly improve the symptoms of dystonia. People with primary dystonia generally have some response to DBS. Those with a known genetic cause seem to improve the most with DBS. However, there are people with primary dystonia who do not respond to DBS, and at this point, we do not know enough to be able to predict who will and who will not respond. Individuals with secondary dystonias are generally not candidates for DBS because they tend not to benefit. The one exception to this rule is tardive dystonia, a form of dystonia caused by exposure to a medication that blocks dopamine. The most common dopamine-blocking agents are antipsychotic medications such as haloperidol (Haldol).

DBS for Dystonia

A 41-year-old woman initially experienced a slow progression of involuntary turning of the head to the left 10 years prior to DBS evaluation, preventing her from looking straight. This was accompanied by pain in her neck. Over the years, the dystonia then spread into her face and eyes, causing forced eye closure and inability to open the eyes for minutes at a time. She worked as a medical receptionist, and her dystonia made it impossible for her to work 3 years before surgery. Multiple medications were tried, without help. Botulinum toxin injections helped initially, but lost effectiveness after 6 years. She was otherwise in good health and had a normal brain scan.

She underwent DBS surgery, where electrodes were placed in the GPi bilaterally. One year after the surgery, she had about a 60% improvement in her symptoms. She no longer had noticeable eye closure or neck pain. While she still had involuntary turning of her head, she was able to keep her head straight if she placed her hand on her chin. These improvements allowed her to work again on a part-time basis.

THREE

Do I Qualify for Surgery?

Now that you know what DBS does and what it can potentially do, the next question you probably want to know is: Am I a candidate for this procedure? Believe it or not, not all physicians (and not even all neurologists) will know the answer to this question. However, knowing the answer to this question is critical to the success of DBS. After all, if you are not a good candidate in the first place, you will likely not have a good outcome. The best way for you to find out if you are a good candidate for DBS is to go to a center where they have a multidisciplinary team that specializes in the evaluation and care of individuals undergoing DBS; finding that team is the topic of Chapter 4. In this chapter, we go over the basics of what makes a good DBS candidate. This may give you an idea of whether or not you might qualify.

PARKINSON'S DISEASE

When to Consider DBS

Because DBS surgery does have risks, it should be offered only when the benefits of the surgery outweigh those risks. Therefore, if you have Parkinson's disease, we are going to start with *when* you should be evaluated for DBS surgery. You should only consider surgery if you have one of the following conditions.

1. You are having motor fluctuations that interfere with activities and cannot be resolved with medication changes.
2. You have a tremor that interferes with activities and is not helped by medications.
3. You cannot tolerate any of the Parkinson's disease medications because of side effects such as nausea or impulse control problems.

If none of these conditions describes you, then you should hold off on getting an evaluation for DBS surgery because you likely will not be considered.

So what do we mean by motor fluctuations? Motor fluctuations occur when you start experiencing wearing off and/or dyskinesias. Remember that, in the last chapter, we talked about levodopa and what can happen with the response to levodopa as Parkinson's disease progresses. Early on in Parkinson's disease, levodopa helps the motor symptoms such as slowness, stiffness, and tremor and frequently lasts from one dose to another, even if a whole night goes by without taking medication. However, as time goes on, the levodopa effect gets shorter and shorter. This is called *wearing off*. As the disease progresses, people living with Parkinson's disease start to depend on the levodopa to function. As they take levodopa, the medication "kicks in," relieves stiffness, and makes movements more fluid, but it only lasts for a short period of time. The cycle then begins again with another dose, and this cycle recurs throughout the waking day, with frequent periods of "on" time followed by frequent "off" times. In addition, in more advanced disease, the "on" times are complicated by *dyskinesias*, the abnormal, involuntary movements that make someone look fidgety. Both dyskinesias and frequent "off" times can interfere with your ability to do things and reduce the quality of your life. DBS can reduce these motor fluctuations potentially for at least 10 years after surgery.

However, many people can delay the need for surgery with adjustments in their medications, so a concerted effort should be made to alter the timing and doses of dopaminergic medications before considering DBS. Below, we list some strategies that can be tried to help wearing off.

1. Adding or increasing the dose of a dopamine agonist (e.g., pramipexole or ropinirole; in countries where available, cabergoline and lisuride may also be used). This class of medications stimulates the dopamine receptors in the brain. They are also longer-acting than levodopa and can make "on" times last longer.
2. Adding a COMT inhibitor such as entacapone or tolcapone. These medications prevent the breakdown of dopamine in the brain, allowing dopamine to hang out for a longer period of time and prolonging "on" times. Tolcapone is associated with liver toxicity, so liver function has to be monitored regularly in individuals taking these medications.

3. Adding an MAO-B inhibitor such as selegiline or rasagiline. Similar to entacapone, these medications can also reduce dopamine breakdown in the brain.
4. Shortening intervals between levodopa doses.
5. Trying apomorphine, an injectable dopamine agonist, for individuals with sudden and unpredictable "off" periods.

Here are some strategies that can be used to help reduce dyskinesias.

1. A trial of amantadine.
2. Reducing the amount of levodopa given per dose and taking it more frequently. For example, if you are taking one full pill of levodopa every 4 hours, but have severe dyskinesias, taking only a one-half pill of levodopa and increasing the frequency to every 2–3 hours may help.
3. If you are taking a sustained or controlled release levodopa preparation, switching to regular release levodopa may help.
4. Increasing the dose of the dopamine agonist and reducing the dose of the levodopa may help.

Please keep in mind that not all strategies can be tried in everyone. You should talk with your neurologist to see if any of these strategies can be employed before considering DBS.

The other two situations we listed that may warrant an evaluation for DBS include a disabling tremor that does not respond to medications and people living with Parkinson's disease who are intolerant of medications because of severe nausea or vomiting, or impulse control problems. Impulse control problems are those in which you get strong urges that you cannot control. Common examples of impulse control problems include gambling, hypersexuality, or compulsive shopping.

If you have a tremor that interferes with activities, you should at least be tried on high doses of levodopa (up to 1500 mg/day) and a medication called trihexyphenidyl, which helps only tremor in Parkinson's disease, before going for DBS evaluation. If you are intolerant to Parkinson's disease medications because of severe nausea, adding extra carbidopa (25 to 100 mg) or domperidone (not available in the U.S.) may help. If you have an impulse control disorder, an effort should be made to wean off your dopamine agonist.

DBS Selection Criteria for Parkinson's Disease

You are a good candidate for DBS if you have:

1. A diagnosis of Parkinson's disease without evidence of an atypical parkinsonian syndrome.
2. A robust and sustained response to levodopa.
3. Presence of complications from chronic levodopa therapy such as dyskinesias, wearing off, and on–off phenomena or, alternatively, a tremor-predominant presentation.
4. Absence of dementia or active psychiatric illnesses such as severe depression.

The most important criterion for consideration of DBS is that you actually have Parkinson's disease. You might think, "Of course I have Parkinson's disease. That's what my doctor told me." However, there are many disorders that mimic Parkinson's disease, and because there is no definitive test, neurologists are only about 80% accurate with the initial diagnosis. These disorders that mimic Parkinson's disease can be difficult to pin down, and neurologists often use terms like atypical Parkinson's disease, atypical parkinsonism, parkinsonism, or a parkinsonian syndrome to characterize these other disorders. Yet, these people are often referred for consideration of DBS.

The atypical parkinsonisms include multiple system atrophy (MSA) and progressive supranuclear palsy (PSP), dementia with Lewy bodies (DLB), and corticobasal degeneration (CBD). One of the main things that distinguish these atypical parkinsonisms from Parkinson's disease is the response to Parkinson's disease medications, specifically levodopa. People with Parkinson's disease respond well to levodopa, whereas people with atypical parkinsonism do not. They are often sent for consideration of DBS because there often are no other treatment options. However, DBS systems have been placed in many individuals with atypical parkinsonism, only to fail. A prominent DBS center in Florida looked at all the individuals that had been referred to their center as "DBS failures" and found that about 12 percent of these people had atypical parkinsonisms that would not be expected to respond to DBS. This is why we recommend that you be evaluated at a center specializing in DBS. These centers have neurologists that specialize in movement disorders such as Parkinson's disease and can confirm that you actually have Parkinson's disease in addition to making sure that you are an appropriate candidate for surgery.

The second criterion for DBS for Parkinson's disease is a robust and sustained response to levodopa. Why? If you have a good response, you are likely to have Parkinson's disease, as mentioned earlier. Additionally, response to levodopa is also one of the best indicators of a good outcome from DBS. Several studies have shown that the improvement you get from DBS is directly related to the amount of improvement you get from levodopa. Furthermore, DBS does not make you better than your medications, which means that your best "on medication" function will be your best "DBS" function. Because DBS is delivered constantly, though, you will feel like you are "on medications" for the entire day.

To evaluate response to levodopa, many centers will conduct an off–on evaluation. This is where you come to the clinic appointment without having taken your Parkinson's disease medications overnight. You are then examined using the Unified Parkinson Disease Rating Scale (UPDRS), which is the most commonly used scale to rate motor symptoms in Parkinson's disease. On the UPDRS, higher scores indicate more impairment. You then take your Parkinson's disease medications, and after they have kicked in, the UPDRS is administered again. In general, most centers use an improvement of at least 30% in the UPDRS score as a benchmark for DBS approval. However, the more you improve on this test, the better a candidate you are.

On the flip side, those features that do not improve with Parkinson's disease medications also will not improve with DBS. Some people may not get offered surgery, even if they have Parkinson's disease and have a response to levodopa, because they are hoping to improve a symptom that does not improve with medication. The most common example is independent walking. Many people have a good response to levodopa, where the levodopa relieves tremor or rigidity and may even cause dyskinesias, but when the medication is working at its best, they still need to use a walker or are wheelchair bound. Unfortunately for these people, DBS will not help them walk independently. If you need a walker when off medications and can walk independently when the medications are working for you, then DBS will help you maintain independent walking. Other features that do not improve with DBS include speech and balance. The one exception to this rule is tremor, which may not respond to levodopa or other Parkinson's disease medications, but responds nicely to stimulation. This is why you should consider DBS if you have a tremor that interferes with activities and is not helped by medications.

The third criterion for selection of appropriate DBS candidates is the presence of motor fluctuations such as dyskinesias or wearing off that cannot be corrected by medication adjustments and interfere with quality of life. We have already mentioned that DBS does not improve your absolute motor function above medications. However, what DBS can do is make you feel like you are in the "on medication" state for longer periods of time. Therefore, instead of fluctuating from off to on to off to on throughout the day, DBS is designed to make you feel like you are "on" the entire day. In addition, if the electrodes are placed in the STN (see Chapter 2 for more information about the different targets), the total dose of medications may be reduced. When levodopa is reduced, there is also less dyskinesia. Therefore, to picture what DBS can do for you, imagine yourself in your "on" medication state all day, without dyskinesias, and you will have an idea of the possibility of DBS. You may also be a candidate for DBS if you have a tremor that does not respond to medications.

The final selection criterion includes the absence of dementia or active psychiatric illness. DBS centers should have potential candidates undergo detailed neuropsychological testing to determine the presence or absence of dementia. Neuropsychological testing generally takes a couple of hours to complete and tests not only your memory but also your ability to pay attention, your language function, your visual–spatial function, and your ability to process information. Preoperative screening for dementia is mandatory because people with dementia may be unable to provide appropriate feedback when the DBS device is tested. This, in turn, may affect the ability of the surgical team to place the DBS electrode in the right place, and definitely would affect the ability of the neurologist or nurse programmer to set the DBS device at the best settings. More importantly, however, cognition in people with Parkinson's disease may worsen after DBS surgery. Long-term studies on people with Parkinson's disease undergoing DBS have shown that mild cognitive decline after surgery is fairly common. Because the cognitive changes are relatively mild, people with no problems in thinking or memory prior to surgery may not notice much difference after surgery. However, those with significant problems in thinking and memory prior to surgery may worsen into a dementia.

In addition, there are reports of people becoming severely depressed after DBS surgery to the point where some even attempt suicide. We still do not know what other factors put people at risk for becoming depressed after surgery other than a previous history of depression. Depression, however, does seem to be more common when electrodes are placed in the STN as opposed to the GPi. The presence of active depression when being evaluated for surgery can also cause significant problems with attention, memory, and executive function, resulting in a neuropsychological evaluation consistent with dementia. These deficits may disappear when the depression is controlled. Thus, if mood is not assessed or improperly evaluated, it may result in the exclusion of candidates who might otherwise be appropriate. Because of this, it makes sense to exclude people with uncontrolled psychiatric illness from having DBS surgery.

OTHER CONSIDERATIONS FOR PARKINSON'S DISEASE

Age

Many people have questions about DBS regarding age. Some surgical centers have been using 70 years of age as a cutoff because early studies demonstrated that people under age 70 tended to show greater motor improvement than people over 70. However, it has also been clearly reported in the medical literature that people over the age of 70 can still have great benefit from DBS. Why younger people have better DBS motor outcomes is not entirely clear, but older people may have more medical problems that increase surgical risk and may take longer to recover from surgery. Older individuals are also more likely to have more problems with thinking and memory. We feel that a strict age requirement for DBS may exclude some good candidates. Thus, potential candidates over the age of 70 should be evaluated on an individual basis. If the DBS center you have chosen has an age cutoff, and you want to be evaluated, you may have to find a different center.

General Health

The entire DBS procedure is a lengthy process. Depending on the center, some individuals can be in the operating room for up to 8 hours or more, in unusually long cases. The surgery is demanding because you have to be awake. For people with Parkinson's, you also have to be off medications during much of the procedure. To tolerate the surgery, it is essential that you be in good general health.

One of the purposes of the DBS evaluation process is to identify problems that put you at high risk for surgery. Medical illnesses that put you at risk of surgical complications, such as uncontrolled high blood pressure, diabetes, or severe cardiopulmonary disease, may cause the DBS team to exclude you from surgery.

Support of Family and Friends

We cannot overemphasize the importance of emotional support from friends, families, or caregivers. After surgery, it can take months to optimize the stimulator settings while adjusting medication. This is a time of constant change, and it may seem like things are not improving or not improving as quickly as you would like. You may also need help around the house or someone to take you to the clinic for the frequent stimulator adjustments. We have seen firsthand how a lack of family support can negatively affect an otherwise successful surgery. See Chapter 5 for more details on getting family and friends involved.

Expectations

DBS surgery cannot be considered successful if your expectations are not met. One of the purposes of this book is to help you have a realistic expectation of the surgical results. If you expect to run a marathon after the surgery when you have never run a marathon in your life, then DBS surgery is never going to be successful. If you understand what the DBS surgery can realistically accomplish, and you are OK with that, then you increase the chances of success.

ESSENTIAL TREMOR

When to Consider DBS

As mentioned in Chapter 2, there are several medications available to treat essential tremor, with propranolol and primidone being the top agents. Many people will respond to medications, but about 30% have no response or minimal response to medications. It obviously does not make sense to opt for DBS when the medications are controlling symptoms. However, what if they do not? It then depends on whether or not the tremors affect your ability to do things and whether you can live with them. You should only consider surgery for essential tremor if:

1. You have tremors that limit your ability to do things.
2. You have tried at least three medications for essential tremor and none of them have worked, or you have had side effects that prevent you from taking higher doses.

The first criterion is somewhat vague because different people have different ideas of when the tremors are limiting. For example, if you were a surgeon, a very mild tremor may limit your ability to perform your job and may force you to consider DBS. However, if you had that same tremor, but had retired from the workplace and it did not interfere with any daily activities such as eating or writing, you may not consider DBS. We once had a person whose job required him to work with explosive chemicals. He had such a mild tremor that it would not have triggered a DBS evaluation in most other people. However, his tremor limited his ability to perform his job because of its very nature, and he underwent DBS surgery. (He did well, by the way, and has not caused any accidental explosions.) Because of the risk of surgical complications, you should only consider DBS if you cannot live with your tremors the way they are.

One of the most common mistakes we see in individuals who have been referred to us is that, although they may have tried several different medications in the past, they may not have taken high-enough doses to see an effect. Therefore, we have listed in a table the common medications used for essential tremor with upper limits of the dose by which we would expect an effect on tremor. If your physician has not prescribed the doses of these medications to the doses listed, you may consider going back to your physician to try higher doses before going for DBS evaluation.

Doses of Essential Tremor Medications

Clonazepam: up to 6 milligrams daily
Gabapentin: up to 2700 milligrams daily
Mirtazepine: up to 45 milligrams daily
Primidone: up to 350 milligrams daily
Propranolol: up to 320 milligrams daily
Topiramate: up to 400 milligrams daily

DBS Selection Criteria for Essential Tremor

Most DBS centers will consider you for DBS if:

1. You have a diagnosis of essential tremor, and your tremors limit or interfere with your activities.
2. You have not responded to high doses of at least three tremor medications.
3. You do not have dementia or active psychiatric illnesses.

Other Considerations for Essential Tremor

The target for essential tremor is the VIM thalamus, which is not as deep as the target for Parkinson's disease. In addition, DBS is usually done only on one side for essential tremor. This cuts down the risks for cognitive decline and other surgical complications. As a result, age is not as much of an exclusion factor for DBS surgery in essential tremor as it is in Parkinson's disease. We would encourage you to read the section Other Considerations for Parkinson's Disease in this chapter, as the subsections on general health, support, and expectations apply to people living with essential tremor as well.

DYSTONIA

When to Consider DBS

If you have dystonia, you should consider DBS when your dystonia interferes with daily activities or your quality of life. Again, the decision as to when the dystonia is severe enough to interfere with your life is an individual one. Furthermore, you should also make sure that there are no other medications that can be tried that could help restore some of that quality of life. Strategies/medications that should be tried include the following.

1. Botulinum toxin. There are many brands of botulinum toxin, including rimabotulinumtoxinB (Myobloc), incobotulinumtoxinA (Xeomin), and abobotulinumtoxinA (Dysport), but the best known of the botulinum toxins is onabotulinumtoxinA (Botox). These medications are injected into the affected muscles and block the signal from the nerve to the muscle. Because the muscles never get the signal to contract, the muscle relaxes and relieves symptoms of dystonia. Unfortunately,

expert injectors of botulinum toxin are not available everywhere. People may not respond to botulinum toxin for a number of reasons, but the most common reasons are that not high enough a dose was injected or that incorrect muscles were targeted. It is also possible that you may be resistant to botulinum toxin. To make sure that you truly do not respond to botulinum toxin, we would recommend that you be evaluated by a movement disorder specialist (a neurologist with specialty training in movement disorders such as Parkinson's disease, essential tremor, and dystonia) with at least 2 years experience injecting for dystonia. There may be a good chance that you might respond to botulinum toxin if it is injected in the correct muscles with the correct doses.

2. Trihexyphenidyl. This is an anticholinergic medication that often helps dystonia, especially in children. Unfortunately, the side effects including sleepiness, dry mouth, urinary retention, and confusion limit its use. Doses greater than 20 mg/day have been shown to be effective in children with dystonia, but in adults, such high doses may not able to be reached because of negative side effects.

3. Benzodiazepines. These are agents commonly used for anxiety but may also help in dystonia. Valium, clonazepam, lorazepam, and alprazolam are the most commonly used medications in this class.

4. Muscle relaxants. In our experience, this class of medication rarely helps dystonia but is still worth a try before considering DBS. Common names for medications in this class include baclofen, cyclobenzaprine, tizanidine, methocarbamol, carisoprodol, and metaxalone.

Please keep in mind that not all strategies can be tried in everyone. You should talk with your neurologist to see if any of these strategies can be employed before considering DBS.

DBS Selection Criteria for Dystonia

The selection criteria for dystonia are not as clear as they are for Parkinson's disease or essential tremor. However, most DBS centers will consider you for DBS if:

1. You have a diagnosis of primary dystonia (can be focal or generalized) or a tardive dystonia.

2. The dystonia causes you to be in pain or to adopt abnormal postures that limit or interfere with your activities.
3. You do not have fixed contractures.
4. You have not responded to medications.
5. You do not have dementia or active psychiatric illnesses.

Primary dystonias are dystonic conditions that either are genetic or do not have another identifiable cause. They can be focal, which means that they affect only one body part, or generalized, which means that they affect the entire body. If you have a secondary dystonia, that means that your dystonia is due to something else, such as a structural lesion in the brain (tumor), a neurodegenerative disease (Huntington's disease), or a number of other causes. Secondary dystonias, in general, do not respond to DBS. The exception is tardive dystonia, which is a secondary dystonia that occurs after long-term exposure to dopamine-blocking agents such as antipsychotics or antinausea medications. Tardive dystonias may respond very well to DBS.

The absence of fixed contractures is important. A contracture is a permanent shortening of muscle, tendon, or scar tissue that produces a deformity, especially around a joint. Contractures can develop in individuals for multiple reasons, but in dystonia, it usually occurs because the joint/limb is not used. Because the contracture results from shortening of a muscle or tendon, or because of scar tissue, and not from abnormal signals in the brain, DBS will not be able to treat contractures.

Other Considerations for Dystonia

Similar to essential tremor, there is no established upper age limit for dystonia. However, because generalized and severe cases of dystonia often occur in children, and children are still growing, implantation of a DBS device has special considerations. First of all, there have been reports of DBS lead migration. That is, after the DBS has been placed in the target, it may lose its effectiveness because the lead moves out of the target as the child grows and matures. Also, many revisions may be needed to place new extension wires as the body gets bigger. The benefits of the surgery should be weighed against these risks in addition to the typical surgical risks that accompany DBS. As people with dystonia are typically younger than people with Parkinson's disease, they are in better general health, but we would encourage you to read the section Other Considerations for Parkinson's Disease regarding family support and expectations.

THE DBS EVALUATION PROCESS

While there are no established requirements for what constitutes a comprehensive DBS evaluation, most DBS centers will have an evaluation process in place. The critical evaluations in this DBS evaluation process regardless of whether you have Parkinson's disease, essential tremor, or dystonia include the following.

1. Evaluation and examination by a movement disorder specialist for the surgery. A movement disorder specialist is a neurologist who specializes in the care of people with Parkinson's disease, essential tremor, or dystonia. The purpose of this visit is to make sure that your diagnosis is correct and that you are an appropriate candidate for DBS. The movement disorder neurologist will perform a complete neurological examination and evaluate mood and cognition as well. Please be aware that the movement disorder specialist may have suggestions for other medications to try before completing the rest of the DBS evaluation. If you have Parkinson's disease, this particular visit may include an off/on medication evaluation using the UPDRS (described earlier). Alternatively, the off/on evaluation may be scheduled separately after you have tried other medications. If you have essential tremor, the severity of your tremors will be rated as you perform tasks with your hands, such as handwriting or drinking from a cup. If you have dystonia, a different rating scale will be used to rate its severity.

2. Evaluation and examination by a neurosurgeon who specializes in DBS surgery. One of the purposes of this visit is to meet the person who will perform the surgery. The neurosurgeon will also confirm the movement disorder specialist's opinion that you are an appropriate candidate and will also evaluate for other factors that might impact the surgery, such as your other medical problems. The risks and benefits of DBS surgery should be discussed with you, and the neurosurgeon should also talk to you about the most appropriate

target in the brain. At this visit, you should ask questions about the surgeon's experience and complication rate.

3. Neuropsychological examination. The purpose of this visit is to make sure that you do not have significant cognitive problems such as dementia. The neuropsychologist will perform a full battery of tests to evaluate your cognition and memory. The effects of mood disorders such as anxiety and depression on cognitive testing will also be looked at. This may last a couple of hours. The test is designed to be extremely difficult, so do not be surprised if you think you failed after you complete the testing.

4. Magnetic resonance imaging (MRI) of the brain. While you may have had MRIs in the past, most centers will repeat brain imaging. This is because there are special sequences that the neurosurgeon needs to plan your surgery and the approach he or she will take.

The above is the minimum that a DBS center will do as part of the evaluation. Some centers will have other evaluations. For example, some may have you see a psychiatrist prior to surgery to make sure you have no active psychiatric problems. Some centers may have individuals undergo a social work evaluation to discuss family and other social support, expectations from the surgery, and insurance issues regarding the surgery. These issues may also be discussed by the neurologist, neurosurgeon, neuropsychologist, or psychiatrist at other centers.

DBS is a big thing to consider. We believe that the best outcomes are seen at a center that conducts a comprehensive evaluation prior to surgery. We have seen people that were just sent to see a neurosurgeon and then underwent surgery a couple of weeks later. Although many of these people did just fine, the ones who had the poorest results seem to have been evaluated in this fashion. If you want to consider DBS and think it is appropriate for you, we would encourage you to seek out a DBS center that specializes in this type of procedure and make sure you feel comfortable with their approach. We tell you how to choose your DBS team in the next chapter.

FOUR

Choosing the Health Care Team that Is Right for You

When considering DBS, one of the most important decisions you will make is your choice of a DBS health care team. Your decision will impact not only you but also your family and other care partners. Undergoing DBS surgery leads to a long-term relationship with those who will manage your DBS system. There will be several visits prior to your surgery. After surgery, you will be followed for as long as you have your DBS. Having the right health care team before and after surgery, as well as for your long-term follow-up, will help to ensure you have the best possible experience. To have a good outcome from your DBS surgery, you need to choose a team that you trust will provide you with excellent care.

Since the approval of DBS for Parkinson's disease, tremor, and dystonia by the FDA, there has been an increase in the number of surgeons performing DBS surgery. It is estimated that there are approximately 250 DBS centers in the USA. You may be referred to one of these centers by your neurologist or primary care physician, or you may get a recommendation through a support group, friend, or a health care worker that you know personally. Your favorite Internet search engine may also be useful in finding information about DBS centers in your area. However, how do you know which centers are qualified to perform DBS surgery? What makes a qualified DBS center? Unfortunately, there is no "certification" process for becoming a DBS center or for surgeons who want to provide this service. Similarly, there is no standardized process for selecting the best candidates for DBS. It will largely be up to you to determine if the DBS center that has been recommended is right for you. In this chapter, we will describe how to find your ideal DBS team.

THE DBS TEAM: CONSIDERATIONS

When choosing a DBS team, you will need to consider where you live and the distance you must travel to the DBS center. There are likely to be several appointments prior to surgery. After surgery, there will be regular follow-up visits. These numerous visits before and after surgery make distance from home an important consideration. Make sure you are prepared to travel back and forth to the DBS center as much as needed. We recommend that you choose a center that is as close to your home as possible.

If you have your DBS surgery a long distance from your home, do not assume that you will be able to find someone closer to home that will take over the management of your DBS after it is implanted. While it may certainly be possible to be followed closer to home, do not wait until after your surgery to find a local DBS physician. It is best to make those arrangements before surgery. Whenever possible, we believe it is best to have your long-term follow-up done by the members of the team that did your preoperative evaluation and DBS surgery. They have insight into your condition and DBS surgery that an outside physician may not be able to appreciate.

It also should not be assumed that the closest center to your home is the best choice for you. While distance is an important factor, there are a number of other considerations to think about when choosing a DBS center. Among the most important factors in choosing a DBS center are the experience and the skill of the health care providers. We strongly believe that the best outcomes are achieved by experienced, well-trained, multidisciplinary DBS teams.

MEMBERS OF THE DBS TEAM

The DBS team is a group of health care providers who work together to help determine if DBS is the right choice for you. They evaluate your condition to determine whether you will benefit from DBS. They also consider any adverse effects that DBS may have on your condition. After surgery, the team provides ongoing management of your DBS.

The DBS team is led by a DBS neurologist and a DBS neurosurgeon. Others on the team may include neuropsychologists or psychiatrists, speech and language pathologists, nurses, nurse practitioners, physician assistants (PAs), neurophysiologists, social workers, and physical therapists. Together, they have the knowledge and experience to care for people with DBS. The following information describes the role and qualifications of the key health care providers that may be on your DBS team. When choosing your DBS team, be sure to ask about their training and experience.

The Neurosurgeon

The neurosurgeon is responsible for placing your DBS system and managing any surgical complications. Careful consideration should be given to the reputation of the neurosurgeon on your DBS team. A neurosurgeon is a physician who has completed 4 years of college, 4 years of medical school, a surgical internship, and 5–6 years of neurosurgery residency. Ask if the neurosurgeon is board-certified by the American Board of Neurological Surgery. Board certification means that the surgeon has met the board requirements for education, peer review, and examination in the practice of neurological surgery.

DBS surgery is a stereotactic procedure that uses images to guide placement of the lead. A qualified DBS neurosurgeon should have undergone specialized training beyond the neurosurgery residency in a fellowship related to stereotactic or functional neurosurgery. This means that the neurosurgeon is specially trained in neurosurgical procedures using computer images to reach precise targets in the brain.

A key element of DBS success is experience. The DBS neurosurgeon should average at least one DBS surgery per month to remain proficient. If the neurosurgeon does not perform very many DBS surgeries, he or she will not have enough experience to maintain his or her skills. This may lead to longer operative times and complications. When meeting the surgeon, ask about the frequency of the DBS surgeries that he or she performs and the number of cases he or she has performed in his or her career. Also, inquire about the rate of complications experienced by the neurosurgeon. Find out how his or her complication rate compares with other DBS centers. No more than 2%–3% of the neurosurgeon's cases should result in serious or permanent complications.

When considering the neurosurgeon, ask about the availability of another qualified neurosurgeon to cover when the DBS neurosurgeon is not available. Inquire about who covers for the DBS neurosurgeon in the off-hours, in the weekends, or when he or she is out of town. Is the covering physician experienced? Is coverage left to a general neurosurgeon, neurosurgery resident, or physician's assistant? The ability to manage complications from DBS surgery is as important as the ability to perform the surgery. If your DBS surgeon is not available, there should be another neurosurgeon available who is equally well trained and experienced.

The neurosurgeon's hospital or medical center affiliation is another important consideration. At minimum, the facility should be accredited by the Joint Commission on Accreditation of Healthcare Organizations (JCAHO). JCAHO focuses on patient safety and the quality of care. Hospitals and health care facilities that meet the standards for JCAHO accreditation provide care using good health care practice and policy. Many third-party insurance payers make JCAHO accreditation a requirement for payment. If the facility is not accredited, your insurance may not cover the DBS procedure at that facility. General information about the accreditation status can be located on the hospital or medical center website. Your insurance carrier will also have information about whether they have a contract with the chosen facility.

Consider the reputation of the health care facility where your DBS surgeon is employed. Does it have a good reputation in the community? Your primary care physician, your insurance company, or someone you know in the health care industry may provide important insight about the care provided at the hospital affiliated with the DBS neurosurgeon. You will want a facility with a surgical suite that houses state-of-the-art technology and image guidance equipment. Is there an MRI suite on site? Information about the available equipment may be described in the hospital or DBS team written literature or Internet website. The neurosurgeon can provide information about the methods and equipment he or she uses for his or her DBS cases. Surgical methods and equipment will be discussed later in this book.

If microelectrode recording is used during surgery, it is *essential* to have an experienced neurophysiologist to accurately interpret the recordings. (See Chapter 7 for more information on the use of microelectrode recording during surgery.) In some DBS centers, the neurophysiologist may also be the DBS neurosurgeon or neurologist. In others, it may be a different member of the team. The neurophysiologist records and interprets electrical activity of the brain. The recordings help precisely locate the target in the brain for placement of the DBS electrode. Some centers do not use microelectrode recordings because they feel confident about their ability to correctly place the DBS lead in the target without them. Some centers may also perform intraoperative MRI rather than microelectrode recordings to confirm placement. Since most centers still use microelectrode recording during surgery, if the center you are considering does not use this, you should ask why.

The Neurologist

While the neurosurgeon manages the surgical placement of DBS, the neurologist provides ongoing follow-up after DBS placement. The DBS neurologist is a physician who has completed medical school, a 4-year neurology residency, as well as a fellowship in movement disorders. This means that the neurologist has spent an extra year or two beyond the standard neurology residency to learn how to take care of people living with movement disorders such as Parkinson's disease, tremor, and dystonia. The DBS neurologist has also spent additional time taking care of and programming individuals with DBS. As with your DBS neurosurgeon, ask if the neurologist is board certified. The governing board for neurologists is the American Board of Psychiatry and Neurology. Board certification means that the neurologist has met the board requirements for education, peer review, and examination in the practice of neurology. There is no additional formal certification at the present time for care of movement disorders or the care of the individuals with DBS.

The roles of the DBS neurologist are to help select the best candidates for DBS and to provide follow-up care for people living with Parkinson's disease, tremor, or dystonia who have undergone DBS placement. The DBS neurologist should know how to perform DBS programming. Many DBS centers have nurses, nurse practitioners, PAs, or others who know how to program the DBS system. Although it is quite helpful and efficient to have others trained in DBS programming, it is important for the DBS neurologist to also be an experienced DBS programmer. The reason for this is that the best outcomes from DBS involve changes not only in stimulation but also in medications. The few months after DBS surgery as stimulation is being applied and medications are being decreased can be challenging. Thus, evaluation and management of DBS outcomes are best accomplished by neurologists with DBS programming skills who have knowledge of the entire picture. Be wary if the neurologist relies solely on others to perform DBS programming. Also, be cautious if the DBS neurologist relies on the representative from the DBS manufacturer to advise him or her on programming the device. These are signs that the DBS center neurologist has little or no experience with DBS.

The Neuropsychologist

Another important member of the DBS team is the neuropsychologist. A neuropsychologist is a licensed psychologist who has completed postdoctoral training in the specialty of neuropsychology. As a result, the neuropsychologist has extensive knowledge of brain structures and brain function. The neuropsychologist on the DBS team has specialized knowledge and experience in the effects of DBS on brain structures. The DBS neuropsychologist evaluates how behaviors such as thinking and memory are affected by DBS. Because DBS can affect cognition, the neuropsychologist's role is to test cognitive skills to make sure there are no significant problems with memory, confusion, or depression prior to DBS. After surgery, the neuropsychologist evaluates the cognitive effects of DBS. If cognitive problems are identified, the neuropsychologist may make recommendations for treatment. When choosing a DBS center, make sure that there is a neuropsychologist on the team with experience in DBS.

Do your Homework!

*L*earn about DBS and find out about the centers you are considering and the individuals who make up that center. Make sure that you choose a DBS center with a multidisciplinary team of health care professionals who have the training, technology, and expertise in DBS.

Other Members of the Team

The three members listed above are essential for a DBS center. There are usually many other members of the team, although the makeup may be different from center to center. Some centers have a DBS psychiatrist. This is a physician who has completed a 4-year residency in psychiatry. The role of the psychiatrist in DBS is to evaluate for the presence of depression prior to surgery and to manage any mood issues that may arise after surgery. Some have a speech-language pathologist as an integral part of the team. A speech-language pathologist evaluates problems that affect communication. Speech-language pathologists have a minimum of a master's degree, have completed 300–400 hours of clinical training, and have undergone testing for licensure or registration. The speech-language pathologist on the DBS team can be involved in the pre-surgical evaluation, as well as follow-up after the DBS is implanted, and may also be present during surgery to evaluate for possible changes in speech and language that might occur when the stimulation is turned on. The DBS center may also have a social worker who is involved in evaluating your living situation, stressors, and other factors that may impact your response and reaction to DBS surgery. The social worker may also be helpful in understanding and managing expectations for the surgery.

There will be other DBS team members who will play an important role in your DBS experience. Nurses and PAs, as well as the clerical staff, will each have a role in your care. When choosing a DBS center, consider how well you are treated before your surgery. This is a good indication of how well you will be treated during and after surgery. For example, are the encounters pleasant? Do they spend sufficient time with you at each encounter? Is the staff able to answer your questions and provide information? Do they appear organized and professional? Consider the ability to communicate with the DBS team. Do they provide a contact person or direct means of reaching them with any questions or concerns? The ability to communicate with the DBS team is critical to your experience.

*L*earn as much as possible about deep brain stimulation before you undergo surgery. Get a second opinion if you have not already. A lot of people get queasy discussing surgery, but the more information you have, the better equipped you will be to make an informed decision. If your doctor is not willing to take the time to discuss the procedure with you, find one who is.

TALKING TO OTHERS

An excellent way to get information about the DBS team is to speak to others who have gone through the surgery and are being followed at the DBS center. The DBS center should be willing to provide you with the contact information of people who have already been through DBS surgery. If they are unable to do this, be cautious about having your surgery there. Be prepared to talk to other people and ask about their impression of the DBS team. Ask about their experience and whether they would recommend the DBS team. Find out if they had any experiences that would keep them from coming back to this center. Share your particular circumstances and ask for an opinion as to whether they believe the center will provide a good experience for you.

As you consider a DBS team, your family, friends, or others may provide you with insight about your choice of a DBS center. Discuss your options with others to weigh the pros and cons of your decision. If you rely on others for transportation, the location of the center may be vital to your decision. On the other hand, even if you rely on others for transportation, the distance of the center may not be a significant factor to them. It is in your best interest to share information about the DBS center with your family, friends, or others that provide support in your health care needs. Their insight may help you evaluate your options so that you can choose a center that is right for you.

Now that you have decided to have DBS surgery, one of the first and most important decisions to make is which DBS center is right for you. Educate yourself about your options by searching the Internet, consulting with your physician, and speaking with family and friends. Talk to the members of the DBS team to find out about their training and experience. Choosing a convenient location that is near your home will make it much easier to travel back and forth from the many visits that will occur before and after surgery. However, to have the best possible outcome from your DBS, you will also want a center that has an experienced well-trained multidisciplinary DBS team. DBS is a complex procedure that requires expert care to optimize the benefits of DBS. It will be up to you to choose a DBS team that you have confidence will deliver the best care possible.

FIVE

Your Social Support Network—
Family and Friends

Making the decision to undergo DBS surgery is a very personal one. You are an individual living with a chronic disease that impacts all aspects of your life. Only you can determine whether it is worth it for you to undergo brain surgery. Yet, you cannot go through DBS surgery alone. You will need assistance and support from others when you have DBS surgery. Your decision to undergo DBS surgery will affect not only you but also your family and friends. In this chapter, you will learn why it is important to tell those in your network of family and friends about your DBS surgery.

As you consider undergoing DBS, you will frequently read or be told that it is important to have a solid network of social support. Having a good support system is important because those with adequate assistance before and after surgery are the best DBS candidates and are likely to have better outcomes than those who do not have good support systems. The stress of deciding whether or not to undergo DBS, of going through the evaluation, and of going through the surgery may also worsen your symptoms. Such uncertainty, anxiety, or stress can be diminished by having adequate levels of social support. Those who live alone or have little support from family and friends may need to rely on assistance from health care providers or agencies for adequate support when undergoing DBS.

Support systems are a network of people such as family and friends who remain close and provide assistance. Support may be provided in various ways. Emotional support, physical support, and even financial support are examples of assistance that may be provided within your support system. We often think of support systems as those immediate family members who help with daily activities. However, support systems may provide a variety of types of support. Emotional support can be provided by offering encouragement and understanding. Physical support occurs when helping with personal care or providing transportation. Financial support may come from social programs or private resources. Your network of support may include your spouse, children, parents, or other family members. Support systems may extend to close friends or neighbors. Support may also be provided by health care agencies or support groups.

Family and friends who are most likely to be affected by your decision to undergo DBS are those closest to you or those who care most about you. Relationships can be challenged during the stress of DBS surgery. It is precisely for that reason that it is important for you, your family, and friends to be well prepared for the events related to DBS.

The marital relationship is one of the most common and most significant social supports. However, the relationship may be strained as the couple faces the challenges of DBS surgery. The roles of each spouse may change, placing more demands on one while increasing dependence in the other. As recovery takes place, there may be another shift toward independence that may leave the care-giving spouse without purpose. Without adequate coping skills or support, these changes can negatively affect the relationship.

To engage your family and friends in the support that you will need for your DBS surgery, they need appropriate information. They need to know what to expect and what is expected from them. Each individual undergoing DBS will have a unique set of circumstances, resulting in individualized needs for help and support. However, there are some common elements that people undergoing DBS surgery should be prepared to share with those who will assist them. The information can be placed into three categories: before surgery, during surgery, and after surgery.

*B*e sure you understand all the risks and benefits of your surgery. This will help others understand why you are opting for DBS and also open the lines of communication.

BEFORE SURGERY

Before surgery, your friends and family should know your goals for DBS and what symptoms you are most interested in improving with DBS. For example, if you have Parkinson's disease, is controlling tremor your main objective? Or is it to smooth out the ups and downs from the medication? If you have essential tremor, do you want the tremor to be gone completely? Or do you just want enough tremor control so that you can bring a fork to your mouth without spilling? If you have dystonia, are you looking for a reduction in uncomfortable spasms? How much improvement in your posture would you like? Your goals should be realistic, and your support system can help with that if they have the information. It is also important for you and them to understand that although DBS can improve symptoms, it is not a cure for your disease.

We recommend that you have someone with you when you undergo your preoperative evaluations. You are likely to undergo several screening evaluations including a baseline evaluation of your movement disorder (please see Chapter 3 for more information). If you have Parkinson's disease, this evaluation will be performed both off and on your medication. You will also see a neuropsychologist where you will have testing to evaluate your thinking and memory. You will be evaluated by the neurosurgeon and undergo an MRI. You may also be seen by a psychiatrist, a speech pathologist, or a social worker. Each one of these evaluations is an opportunity for you and your family or care partner to be provided information and to ask questions. Because there will be an extensive amount of information provided, we recommend that your spouse, family, or care partner accompany you to each of these visits. Someone else may hear information that you do not hear or remember information that you forget. Someone else may ask questions that you may forget to ask. Be aware that the evaluation process is not only for the DBS team to evaluate you but also an opportunity for you to evaluate the DBS center. The time and care the DBS team takes to answer your questions and those of your family and friends are a reflection of how the DBS team may take care of you during and after the surgery.

Those who plan on accompanying you need to know the purpose of the visits and what to expect at each visit. To provide you with support and help you hear information being provided, they should accompany you into the exam rooms. Having them sit in the waiting room defeats the purpose of having them accompany you to these visits. Have them bring a notepad or pencil and paper so that they can take notes for you. Their input may also be useful. They may be asked to provide or confirm information about your medical status. As you tell your family or friends about the preoperative evaluations, make sure that they are told how long each visit will last. In the event there is waiting time, or if the visits take longer than expected, they should be prepared to bring a book, magazine, coffee, or snack.

DURING THE SURGERY

Your friends and family should be given information about the surgical procedure (see Chapters 6 and 7 for more detailed information). Important points that they need to know include where the surgery will take place, how long the surgery will take, and how long you will be in the hospital.

You will need someone to be at the hospital while you have your surgery. Please make sure that you know ahead of time where you are supposed to report on the day of your surgery. Also, make sure that you know where to park and how to get to the preoperative area. It may even be helpful to do a dry run the day before surgery so that you are not stressed trying to find the right place on the day of surgery. Being prepared will help you to focus on you.

The length of time that you will need someone to stay with you depends on how well you tolerate the surgery. Please see Chapter 7 for more details on the surgery itself. Some centers put all the hardware in on one day. Some place the leads in on one day and then place the extension wire and stimulator in a few weeks later. Let your family and friends know that they do not necessarily have to stay in the surgical waiting room the entire time you are in surgery. Sometimes they can leave their cell phone number with the staff at the reception desk in the surgical waiting area and ask to be contacted with any news, especially if they need to go outside the hospital. Many hospitals may not allow cell phone use within their premises, so as an alternative, some hospitals will give you a pager that will periodically update you on the progression of the surgery or ask you to come to the desk. Additionally, make sure that the family members or friends who accompany you on the day of surgery bring lots of things to do. Some hospitals now have Wi-Fi capability so that your friends and family can bring laptops, iPads, or other favorite gadgets to pass the time.

After lead placement, most people usually stay in the hospital for at least a night. If you feel more comfortable having someone stay with you throughout the night, that can be accommodated, but most hospitals will let only one family member stay. Many hospitals also have rules regarding visitors, especially after 9 or 10 p.m., so make sure you know what the policy is before your surgery. By knowing and sharing this information with your family or friends, you can begin to develop a plan so that there will be adequate assistance in place when you have surgery.

AFTER THE SURGERY

Upon your discharge, you will need someone to drive you home. For safety precautions, we tell people not to drive for 2 weeks after brain surgery. Thus, you will also need someone to stay with you and help you after surgery. Share information about the potential side effects with this person so that he or she feels comfortable and knows what to expect after surgery. Your friends and family should not assume that just because your DBS was implanted, your symptoms will be improved. Although some may have what is called a "honeymoon period," where the symptoms of Parkinson's disease, essential tremor, or dystonia are better immediately after surgery, this improvement is short lived, and your condition returns to its baseline after a few days to a couple of weeks. Then comes the process of turning on your stimulator and increasing it slowly until your symptoms are controlled. In fact, it may take up to 6 months after surgery before your stimulator adequately controls your symptoms.

Friends and family also need to know about your limitations after surgery. In addition to avoiding driving, you will be given a list of instructions for taking medications, caring for your incisions, and activity limitations. This information needs to be shared with your family and friends so that they are in a position to provide appropriate assistance after your surgery.

You are likely to have several programming appointments after your surgery. Your friends and family need to be prepared to continue supporting you during this time. After surgery, during the period when you are being reprogrammed, it is possible to experience side effects or worsened symptoms that may interfere with your ability to perform your daily activities. This is important information to share with your family and friends so that they are prepared to help you as needed.

Although the choice to undergo DBS is a personal decision, going through the preoperative evaluations, undergoing surgery, and recovering from the procedure all require assistance from your family and friends. You will need to identify a network of family or friends that are willing to help you through the experience. In order for them to help, it is necessary to tell your family and friends about the details of the presurgical evaluations, the surgical procedure, and the postoperative recovery. Share your information resources and any other written materials with them.

You will need to be prepared for the reaction of those you tell about the surgery. Not everyone is comfortable listening to detailed information about surgery, so do not take it personally. You may encounter those who believe DBS is too risky, or they may not think your symptoms are bad enough to warrant brain surgery. Under those circumstances, you will need to help them understand your motives for surgery. This may be stressful, which may increase your own fears and anxiety. However, by telling friends and family about your DBS surgery, you can identify a supportive network of those who will assist you along your DBS journey. Good communication between you, your family, and friends is critical to a successful DBS outcome.

SIX

How to Prepare for the Big Day

Y ou have been thoroughly evaluated and are considered to be an excellent candidate for DBS surgery. After considering your options, you have elected to undergo surgery. Your date of surgery is drawing near, and the reality of having DBS surgery is setting in. You may be experiencing mixed emotions of excitement and apprehension. These are normal feelings. After experiencing weeks of uncertainty about whether DBS is right for you, there is relief in knowing the outcome of all those evaluations. However, now you are faced with a new challenge: preparing yourself for DBS surgery. Anxiety, fear, and apprehension are best controlled by having the right information at hand and planning for the big day.

PLANNING FOR THE BIG DAY

Planning for the big day should begin as soon as you are scheduled for surgery. Your support network of family or friends needs to be informed of the date or dates of surgery. Make sure you plan to have a person that will drive you to the hospital and bring you home. After you are discharged to home, you will have some fatigue, as well as discomfort at the surgical incisions. You will have activity limitations placed such as avoiding driving, lifting, or exaggerated movements. You should plan on having someone stay with you for the first few days after surgery to help you manage until you are able to resume your normal activities. If you have children or pets, you will need to make sure you have help in caring for them.

How Much Time Should I Take Off Work?

Plans to take off work should be considered for you, as well as anyone who will be helping you after your surgery. It is best that you and your care partners apply for the appropriate vacation days, sick days, or Family Medical Leave Act as soon as you have a date of surgery. Depending on your response to surgery, you should plan on staying off work for at least 2 weeks after surgery. If your surgeon schedules more than one surgery to place your DBS, you may need to be absent from work up to 8 weeks. Ask your DBS team about the expected length of time you should plan on being absent from work. It is better to plan for more time off work than you need. You can always go back sooner if you recover more quickly.

Insurance and Financial Concerns

Ask yourself if you have the financial resources you need before and after your surgery. DBS is covered by most health insurance plans. However, you may be responsible for a percentage of the cost. Make sure you understand your financial obligation for the cost of your DBS surgery. Your DBS team or hospital accounting department should be able to help with that. Besides the cost of surgery, there are other financial considerations when planning for surgery. Do you have access to reliable transportation and money for gas? Do you have money for any prescriptions or copays that you may need after your surgery? Can you afford to buy groceries if you are off work for a few weeks? Many people face financial struggles on a daily basis. However, having financial concerns as you go through DBS surgery places an added burden and will lead to more stress and anxiety. We recommend that you plan ahead so that you do not have to worry about your finances while you are undergoing DBS surgery. Ask to speak to a social worker to discuss any concerns you may have about your financial situation.

Anxiety

DBS surgery is performed while you are awake. The surgery can provoke anxiety, which may interfere with your ability to get through the surgery. You need to be able to cooperate and provide information during the surgery. If your anxiety interferes with your ability to focus and cooperate during surgery, the procedure will not have a good outcome or may need to be stopped before it is completed. Now is the time to begin planning strategies to overcome your anxiety during surgery. It takes practice to learn effective breathing or other relaxation strategies. Your DBS team may have CDs that you can use at home to practice breathing and relaxation techniques. If you believe listening to music will provide distraction enough to keep you relaxed during surgery, plan ahead on the type of music that works best and ask about using a CD player or iPod with headphones in the operating room. Once you are scheduled for surgery, talk to your DBS team about developing coping strategies so that you become comfortable and skilled using the selected relaxation methods well ahead of your DBS surgery. Controlling your anxiety during surgery is essential for a good outcome.

Daily relaxation strategies will lower anxiety and improve your ability to cope with surgery and recovery. There are books and CDs available at the library and at bookstores that can help you prepare your mind for surgery. However, if you have poorly managed anxiety, depression, or other psychological illness, you should be treated by a psychiatrist prior to DBS surgery.

General Health and Attitude

As your surgery date approaches, you will want to take measures to ensure you are as healthy as possible. The best recovery *after* surgery occurs when you are as healthy as possible *before* surgery. When preparing for surgery, take care of both the physical and mental aspects of improving your health. Mental aspects include improving your attitude and beliefs. Empower yourself by taking steps to cultivate a positive attitude about your upcoming DBS surgery. Eliminate negative thoughts and avoid words such as "can't," "hope," and "try." Replace any negative thoughts with more positive thoughts. This can be done by using words such as "can," "will," and "do." You are more likely to accomplish your goals for DBS if you have a positive attitude.

It has been reported that those with strong spiritual habits such as prayer or meditation enjoy better health and happiness. If your spiritual strength comes from your religion, consult with your clergy for ways to improve your spiritual health prior to surgery. You may find that your mental health benefits from a plan of daily prayers or meditation.

Physical aspects of becoming healthy before your surgery include good nutrition, weight control, and exercise. Choosing a well-balanced diet that includes plenty of fruits, vegetables, and whole grains promotes good health and healing. A well-balanced diet is also important for good bowel health, which is particularly important after surgery. Reduction of unnecessary weight decreases your surgical risks and makes your recovery easier. Daily exercise is also important for improving your health before surgery. Walking, cycling, and swimming are excellent forms of exercise. Unfortunately, many of those who are preparing for DBS surgery have movement disorders that make such exercises difficult. However, any activity or exercise done on a daily basis helps facilitate good health. Ask your physician to recommend exercises that are best for you.

Surgical Clearance—A Clean Bill of Health

Prior to undergoing any surgery, you will need to obtain surgical clearance. This simply means that you will undergo a physical to make sure that you are healthy enough to have surgery. The physical is done within a few weeks of your surgery and may include routine blood tests and electrocardiogram (EKG). It is rare that you would require a blood transfusion; however, you may still have a blood type and screen drawn. Chest X-ray or other tests may be necessary, depending on your health condition. It is important to let your doctor know of any nonhealing wounds or infections. If you have chronic conditions such as heart or kidney disease, you may be asked to also obtain clearance from your specialty physician.

THE DAY BEFORE SURGERY

Medications

Prior to surgery, you will be given instructions about how to take your medications. There are some medications that you must avoid taking prior to surgery. Herbal supplements and some over-the-counter medications can lead to increased bleeding or other adverse effects during your surgery or recovery. We usually recommend that herbal and most over-the-counter products be stopped 2–3 weeks prior to surgery. Medications that contain aspirin, ibuprofen, or other nonsteroidal anti-inflammatory drugs may increase your risk for bleeding. We recommend they be avoided at least 1 week prior to surgery. It is best to provide a current list of all the medications you are taking, including any over-the-counter medications, so that your physician or nurse can give you instructions for each medication.

Those with Parkinson's disease will be given specific instruction about taking Parkinson's disease medications. Most DBS centers perform DBS surgery when individuals are "off" medication. You will likely be instructed to stop your Parkinson's disease medication the night before surgery. Make sure you provide them with a current list of your Parkinson's disease medications so that your DBS team can tell you when to take or stop each of these medications. Some Parkinson's disease medications are long-acting. These usually have the letters CR (controlled release), SR (sustained release), or XL (extended length) after it. These long-acting medications may need to be stopped more than just the night before surgery. In addition, MAO-B inhibitors such as rasagiline and selegilene should be stopped 2 weeks before surgery. You may be asked to bring your medications in their original bottles to the hospital. At minimum, you will be asked to bring a current list of your medications to the hospital, with information about dosage and frequency.

Other Concerns

Make sure you have information about the location of your surgery. If your DBS center is part of a large medical center, your surgery may take place in a location that you are not familiar with. You may find it helpful to familiarize yourself with the location of your surgery ahead of time, so that finding the location does not increase your anxiety on the day of your DBS surgery. If you plan to stay at a hotel near the hospital prior to surgery, it is best to make reservations as far in advance as possible. If you need help locating a hotel near the hospital, ask the DBS team for a recommendation. They should be able to provide you with options and the appropriate contact information for planning your overnight stay.

On the day before surgery, keep your meals light. This will help avoid any gastrointestinal distress that may occur during surgery due to stress or anxiety. On the night before surgery, you will not be able to eat or drink any food or liquids. Avoiding food and drink after midnight makes it less likely for you to have nausea, vomiting, or other complications from having food in your stomach at the time of surgery. There is a risk of experiencing aspiration pneumonia if you vomit food from your stomach.

To reduce the risk of infection, it may be recommended that you take a shower the night before your surgery, as well as in the morning of your surgery. This eliminates much of the bacteria found normally on the skin. Eliminating the bacteria may help reduce the risk of infecting your DBS.

Although serious complications are rare, you should bring a list of your family or friends, with their contact information, or anyone that you would want to have contacted in case of emergency. If you have advance directives such as a Durable Power of Attorney for Health Care, or a Living Will, bring a copy to the hospital so that the document can be placed in your record. In the event of an emergency or significant complication, these documents will ensure that your health care wishes are respected.

Now that the big day has become a reality, you need to prepare yourself for surgery. As your date of surgery draws near, you are likely to feel excitement as well as apprehension. Develop strategies to reduce your anxiety and become as healthy as possible. As you prepare for surgery, make a list of things you need to do so that you are organized. Read and follow the instructions you are given about avoiding or taking medication before surgery. Make sure you get a good night's sleep the night before. Being organized, having the right kinds of information, and planning ahead are the best strategies for preparing for surgery.

SEVEN

What Should I Expect during the Surgery?

Deep brain stimulation (DBS) surgery generally takes place in two stages. In the first stage, the DBS leads are placed into the target locations in the brain. In the second stage, the implanted leads are connected to the stimulator or the implantable pulse generator (IPG). Depending on available resources and the preferences of the neurosurgeon, each DBS team performs the surgery differently.

For example, at some centers, both stages are performed on the same day, making the DBS procedure into a single, long operation. At the other extreme, some centers will implant one lead at a time and one stimulator per side at a time, for a total of four separate operations. Each approach has its advantages and disadvantages. The advantage of having everything done in one operation is that you have fewer operations, which reduces risk of infection and side effects from anesthesia. On the other hand, having everything done in a single operation means that it takes much longer to complete on that day. It makes for a much more complex procedure.

In this chapter, we describe a staged DBS surgery where stage I (lead implantation) occurs first, followed by stage II (placement of the extension wire and stimulator). Stages I and II are separated by some period of time, ranging from a week to several weeks. This approach is between the two extremes listed above and is done at many centers. Thus, for people living with Parkinson's disease or dystonia, two DBS leads would be placed during stage I, one on each side of the brain, followed by stage II later. For essential tremor, a unilateral lead would be placed on the side of the brain opposite the dominant hand in stage I, and then followed by stage II some time later. The advantage to performing surgery in a staged manner like this is that the procedure tends to be tolerated better.

STAGE I: IMPLANTATION OF DBS LEADS

Frame Placement

On the day of surgery, you will start in the preoperative area. You will be asked to remove your clothing, jewelry, and other personal items and change into a hospital gown. An intravenous (IV) line will be placed in your vein so that medications can be administered during surgery. Many centers try to avoid placing a urinary catheter during this part of the surgery. Because you are typically awake during stage I, you will be able to use a bedpan or urinal if needed. However, because you have not been able to eat or drink for several hours, there is usually little concern for your bladder.

The first step in the implantation of the DBS leads is the placement of a lightweight metal frame that looks like a hollow cube. You will be seated comfortably and facing forward. The frame is then fixed to the skull and held in position by four screws, two in the front and two in the back. Numbing medication is injected into the

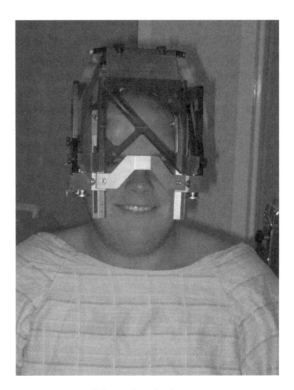

Stereotactic frame

skin at four points where the frame will be fixed to the skull. When the frame is applied, you may feel pressure from the screws, but not pain, due to the numbing medication. If you complain of some pain, then more numbing medication is given. The sense of pressure that people feel can be initially significant but goes away entirely within 5–10 minutes. With the frame placed, you are then taken to the MRI scanner. The MRI uses magnetic fields to take clear and detailed pictures of the brain.

Keep in mind that some centers may do "frameless" surgery. Although not technically frameless, this technique uses a much smaller frame. Rather than looking like a hollow cube that goes around your entire head, the "frameless" approach uses either a small frame that looks like a tripod and is screwed to the top of the skull or another small frame that attaches to the hole drilled in the skull. The approach that your neurosurgeon takes is generally based on his or her training and experience. Neither approach is clearly better than the other. What is important is that your neurosurgeon is experienced with one of the approaches.

Pre-operative MRI

Before entering the MRI, two additional components are attached to the frame: a localizer and an orientation adapter. The localizer includes a fluid-filled chamber that contains a solution that can be seen on the MRI scan. The orientation adapter holds the individual and the frame in good position during the MRI scan. This preoperative MRI scan takes about 10 minutes to perform.

Choosing the Target

The MRI allows the neurosurgeon to see all of the structures in the brain. The neurosurgeon uses this picture to mark the structure where the DBS lead will be placed and determines the path that the electrode shall take from the skull surface to the deep brain target. You are given an intravenous dye prior to the MRI scan, which allows the neurosurgeon to avoid important blood vessels when planning the path of the electrode and thus reduce complications.

The MRI-visible solution in the localizer component allows a unique set of coordinates to be assigned to each location in the brain. By examining the MRI scan, the neurosurgeon can estimate the location of any of the targeted structures such as the subthalmic nucleus (STN), thalamus, or globus pallidus interna (GPi) and associate it with a set of X, Y, and Z coordinates. This allows the surgeon to accurately determine where to place the tip of the lead.

In addition to determining the coordinates of each target, the neurosurgeon also determines the location of the small hole where the DBS electrode can most safely enter the skull. The straight-line trajectory from the skull to the DBS target determines where entry holes may be made safely. The neurosurgeon must take great care to ensure that the trajectory does not cross any blood vessels or other important brain structures. With the targets calculated and the entry locations determined, the operation may now proceed.

Going to the Operating Room

After the MRI is completed, you will be taken from the MRI scanner to the operating room. Once you are in the operating room, you may find it noisy and quite busy with staff preparing for the procedure. Your comfort is important to the neurosurgeon and staff. If you feel discomfort, you should let your surgeon know so that steps can be taken to alleviate any pain or discomfort. Also, if you find the room too cold, ask for additional blankets. Ask if headphones and a CD player or iPod are available for listening to your favorite music or relaxation message.

You will be positioned comfortably on the operating table, and the operating room staff will make sure that the table is well-padded so that you will not be sore. Additional padding may be used to be sure that your back and neck are comfortable. The frame that is fixed to your skull will be secured to the operating table so that it cannot move during the procedure. The head of the bed is raised slightly, so that you will be able to look forward. You will not be able to move your head because it is secured to the table (but you would not want to anyway, since moving your head would alter the path of the electrode and you would risk having the DBS lead placed incorrectly). However, you will be able to freely move your arms and legs.

A narrow strip of hair, just above the forehead (and behind the hairline), is then shaved. It should be noted that the amount of hair shaved differs from center to center. Some neurosurgeons will shave the entire skull, whereas others will shave only a small area. If you care about how much hair is shaved off, you should ask about this before the surgery. The skin is cleansed thoroughly with antibacterial solution to prevent infection. Once the solution dries, sterile drapes are placed to cover the surgical area and to form a bacteria-proof shield. Numbing medicine is then injected into the area where the incision is to be made. Once the incision is made, the targeting apparatus of the frame is used to mark the location on the skull where the small holes are to be made.

Each hole for each DBS electrode is fashioned with a very special drill. The drill is designed to cut through the bone without cutting through any softer tissues than the bone. Because of this feature, the hole can be made in the skull without injuring the brain or its coverings. Because sound conducts well in the bone and earplugs only block sound conducted in the air, the sound of the drill is quite loud for the person undergoing surgery. Some people are also bothered by the vibration or chatter of their teeth from the drill. Because of these two factors, many people say that the drilling is the worst part of the entire procedure. If the vibration is bothersome, ask for a small cloth to hold in your mouth briefly until the drilling is complete. Fortunately, the drilling itself lasts only for a few seconds. The size of the drill hole is about the width of a dime.

Once the drilling is completed, the neurosurgeon attaches the targeting mechanism, which is shaped like a semicircular arc, to the frame. The targeting arc is set to guide the electrode to the intended target coordinates along the planned trajectory. An X-ray may be taken to double-check that the electrode trajectory is accurate.

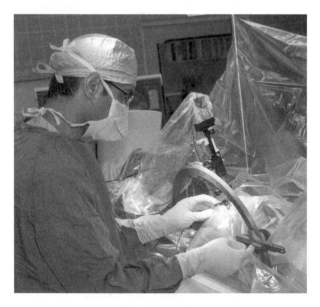

Arc assembly

Electrophysiological (Microelectrode) Recording

Electrophysiological or microelectrode recording is a technology that allows the neurosurgeon, often working with a neurologist or neurophysiologist, to measure the activity of brain cells. By looking at the activity of cells, the neurosurgeon can often determine where the cells are located. Imagine yourself taking a road trip from Detroit down to Miami. If you keep the radio on, you might hear the sounds of Motown when you start the trip. As you drive past Nashville, you probably will start to hear country music on the radio. When you get into Miami, you might hear more Cuban music. The cells of the thalamus, STN, and GPi regions all have very distinct firing patterns, just like Detroit, Nashville, and Miami have different music playing on their radio stations. By measuring the activities of cells, the neurosurgeon can determine the optimal location for the tip of the DBS lead along the trajectory and confirm that the lead is being placed in the correct area.

The electrodes used to examine the firing patterns of brain cells are very fine. In fact, the tips of these electrodes are twenty-five times narrower than the tip of the DBS electrode itself. The use of electrophysiological or microelectrode recording, therefore, allows the optimal DBS electrode target to be found without having to test multiple areas by passing the large DBS electrode into the brain. There is no sensation as the leads are passed through the brain, so there is no discomfort from placement of the electrode.

Placement and Testing of Leads

Once the optimized target location is determined, the DBS lead is placed into the brain. The placement of the lead is confirmed by X-ray. After that, the DBS lead will be turned on and you will be examined. The purpose of this is to make sure that the DBS system can improve symptoms. It also allows the DBS team to test for side effects. When the DBS system is turned on in the operating room, you may feel tingling sensations or mild electrical shocks in the face, arm, or leg opposite the side of the DBS lead. Depending on the location of the lead and the contact being tested, you may see a burst of light, experience double vision, or even feel hot and sweaty. Sometimes you may even feel that the muscles in your face, arm, or leg are spasming. Typically, these side effects will occur only at higher settings. If side effects occur at low settings, the DBS lead may be slightly off and may need to be replaced. If you have ET,

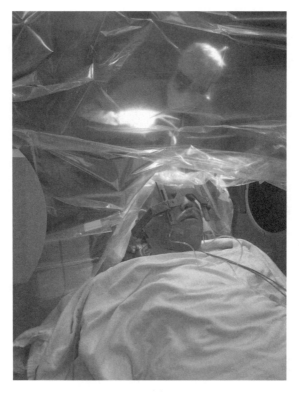

Getting an X-ray in the operating room

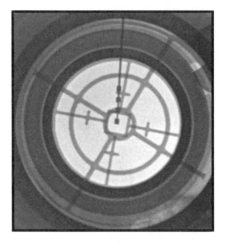

Lead verification

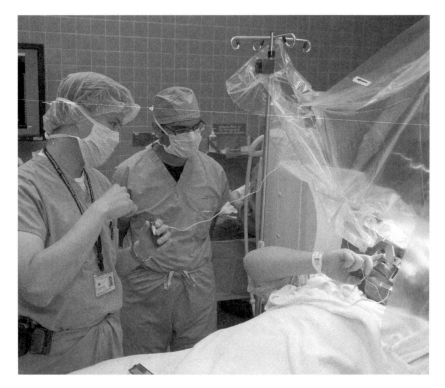

Patient testing

the DBS team will see if the stimulation can help stop your tremor. If you have Parkinson's disease, the DBS team will look at whether stimulation will help tremor (if you have it), relieve stiffness, or improve slowness. You may be asked to write, drink, repeat words or phrases, or move the arms or legs, depending on what your symptoms are. For dystonia, unfortunately, improvement in the posture and pain is usually not seen in the operating room. However, the DBS team can confirm if it is in the correct place based on the side effects you get when the stimulation is turned on.

At some centers, the neurosurgeon and neurophysiologist do the testing. At others, the DBS neurologist is called into the operating room to perform the testing. Some centers may also have a speech-language pathologist present during testing to make sure that there are no speech problems with the stimulator turned on. After testing, the members of the DBS team will come together in the room to discuss whether the lead is appropriately placed or whether adjustments need to be made.

At this point, if you have essential tremor, the bulk of the surgery is over, and you only need to wait for the surgeon to secure the lead to the skull and close the incision before you are taken to the postoperative care unit. However, if you have Parkinson's or dystonia, the electrophysiological recording and DBS lead placement and testing are repeated on the other side of the head. Once both leads are placed, each is secured into its location with a plastic locking cap that fits into the hole drilled in the skull. This cap remains under the skin. As a result, your scalp will feel irregular or "lumpy." This is normal. Your hair will cover the irregularity so that it is not noticeable (unless you have a bald head). The DBS electrodes are placed under the skin, just above the ear. The scalp incision is then closed with surgical staples or sutures. There may be mild pain from the incision at this time, which is easily managed with pain medication. People also often have a headache and feel tired after surgery. Some people will notice swelling at the forehead and under or around their eyes, and there may also be bruising of the soft tissue on the face. This is normal and will subside over the next few days.

DBS Lead Placement Using Intraoperative MRI

A new technique for placement of DBS leads is using intraoperative MRI. This is only being performed at a few select centers thus far. Instead of being placed in a traditional stereotactic frame (the "hollow cube" mentioned earlier), an "aiming device" is applied to the top of the skull that allows the neurosurgeon to get X, Y, and Z coordinates for each part of the brain. Individuals are placed under general anesthesia, and the procedure is done in the radiology suite, not the operating room. The target structure is seen using MRI after the holes are drilled, and the placement of the lead is confirmed with the MRI before closing the incision. All of the instruments and hardware developed for this technique are MRI compatible. No electrophysiological recording or clinical testing is done with this method. The advantages are that the surgery can be done more quickly and can be done under general anesthesia. However, this method is not yet being used at all centers, and the success of the surgery depends on the quality of the pictures obtained by the MRI.

Recovery and Post-operative Imaging

Once the leads are secured in position and the incision is closed, you will be taken to the recovery room. Before that, however, you

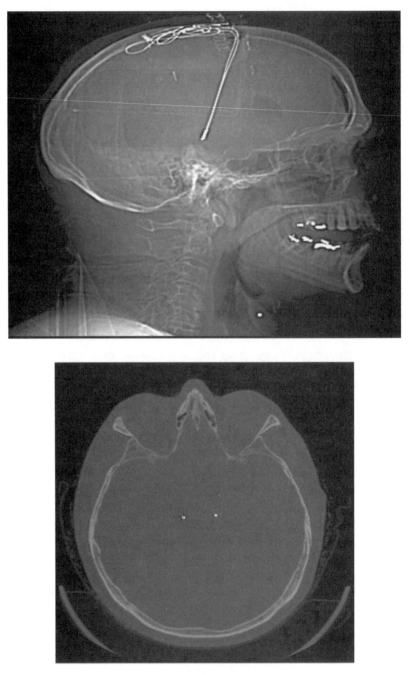

Postoperative CT scan

may be taken to get a postoperative computed tomography (CT) scan to verify the location of the leads and to confirm that there is no abnormal bleeding due to the lead placement. The CT scan does not take as long as an MRI and is not as clear, but is a much better way of detecting blood in the brain. Sometimes this CT may be done after a short wait in the recovery room and before being taken up to your hospital bed.

After surgery, you may be placed in the intensive care unit or in a regular unit. It is typical for most people to be discharged from the hospital on the day after lead placement. When you are discharged to home, you will be given instructions about care of your incisions, pain management, and activity limitations. Those living with Parkinson's disease will likely resume their regular medications, but it is possible that less medication will be needed. Make sure you have someone who will stay with you for a few days until it is certain you have no untoward effects from surgery.

During your hospital stay, you may be surprised that the staff often knows little about the management of movement disorders, especially Parkinson's disease. That is because people with movement disorders are rarely hospitalized for their disease. If you have Parkinson's, you may find that nurses are not as responsive to your need to take your medication promptly, and your medication schedule may be altered. Because the hospital formulary may not have your particular medications available, you may be prescribed different medication than you take at home. To reduce some of the problems related to changes in your medication regimen, we recommend that you bring an accurate list of your medications with the dose and frequency. Your friends and family who are going to support you will need to be your advocate at this time. They (or you) should provide the nurse on each shift a brief educational summary about your condition, especially how alterations in your medications impact your ability to move and function. You should also monitor the administration of your medications, and question any medications you do not normally take. Being proactive about these issues will help make your hospital stay a more comfortable one.

STAGE II: PLACEMENT OF THE STIMULATOR

Stage II is an outpatient procedure in which the stimulator or implantable pulse generator is placed under the skin in the chest and is connected by wires under the skin to the earlier implanted DBS lead. The second stage of DBS surgery may be scheduled anywhere from the next day to several weeks after the first stage, depending on the DBS center. One of the advantages to waiting longer in between stages is that it allows adequate time for the wounds to heal and to ensure that there are no signs of infection from the lead-placement surgery. However, performing stage II closer to stage I may be more efficient in terms of recovery time. Regardless of the interval between lead placement and placement of the stimulator or IPG, it is recommended that there be at least 4 weeks between placement of the lead and initial programming of the stimulator.

Unlike stage I where the individual is awake, stage II is performed under general anesthesia. In other words, you will be completely knocked out. After the anesthesia kicks in, you will be moved to the operating room and placed on the operating table. After cleaning the skin and washing the head with antiseptic solution, a small incision is made over the location where the electrodes are buried under the scalp. The electrodes are then brought to the surface, where they can be accessed.

The neurosurgeon then creates a pocket under the skin, just below the collarbone. This pocket is large enough to hold the stimulator or IPG snugly. Once the pocket is made, the neurosurgeon creates a tunnel under the skin from the pocket, up the side of the neck, and behind the ear to the location where the electrode was buried, using a special tunneling device. Through this tunnel, an extension wire is passed and connected to the DBS electrode on one end and the stimulator on the other. The stimulator is then tested to make sure that it is working properly and is connected correctly to each DBS electrode. The incisions are then closed with sutures. All parts of the DBS system are internal, and nothing is outside of the skin.

For stage II, most people are able to go home as soon as they wake up from surgery. Prescriptions for oral pain medications will be given to help make you comfortable. Rarely, the pain is so intolerable that a person will need to be admitted for further observation. Again, make sure that you have someone with you for this surgery who will be able to drive you home. We also recommend that someone stay with you for a few days after surgery to make sure there are no complications.

EIGHT

I Had the Surgery. Now What?

*A*t this point, you have been through what most people consider the most nerve-wracking part of DBS. However, it is important to remember that the first few months after surgery are equally important. This is when your neurologist or DBS nurse programmer will turn on your stimulators and slowly adjust the settings to help your condition. In some cases, it will not take long to find settings that will help your symptoms; in other cases, it may take a while. We usually tell people that it may take 3–6 months to arrive at a setting that is optimal for them, although in many cases, it does not take as long. During this time period, it may be frustrating to have gone through the surgery and not see immediate results. Keep in mind all that you have been through, and it will be worth it in the end.

THE HONEYMOON PERIOD

The time period right after the leads are placed and before the day of initial programming is sometimes called "the honeymoon period." This is because some people notice an improvement in their symptoms after the surgery with the stimulator turned off, and it may last from a couple of days to a couple of weeks. If you have essential tremor, you may notice that your tremor is less or even gone for this period of time before coming back. People living with Parkinson's may notice less tremor and stiffness, and they are able to move around more fluidly. In medical terms, this is called a "microlesioning effect" and is believed to be due to swelling in the brain that comes from placing the lead. However, it is important to remember that as the swelling goes down and your brain returns to its baseline, the symptoms almost always come back. Because no one can predict how long the honeymoon period lasts, it is important not to stop your medications suddenly, or else you might crash when the effect wears off. Always call your DBS team or neurologist if you have questions about whether you should adjust your medications after surgery.

It is also important to remember that the microlesioning effect does not happen to everyone. Whether you have a microlesioning effect or not does not influence whether the stimulator will work for you when it is turned on. We have operated on many people who did not experience such an effect, but are completely happy with their symptom control from their device.

WHEN IS THE STIMULATOR TURNED ON?

A common question is when the device will be turned on. While the DBS lead in your brain may be tested in the operating room, the stimulator is typically not turned on for some time after the surgery. This practice varies worldwide, with some DBS centers starting programming the day after surgery, and some waiting as long as 60 days. A North American survey of DBS centers published in 2005 found that initial activation of the electrodes took place about 18 ± 12 days after the leads were placed.

Of course, part of this variation depends on how the leads are initially placed. For people with essential tremor who only have one lead placed, 2–4 weeks from lead placement is a good estimate of when the initial programming will start. However, for people with Parkinson's and dystonia who typically have leads placed on both sides of the brain, the start of programming depends on whether the leads are placed simultaneously or whether the second lead is implanted some time after the first side. About half of DBS centers in North America place both leads at the same time. At DBS centers where the leads are placed in each side of the brain in separate surgeries, the second lead is placed about 3–4 months after the first side. Some centers may wait for both sides to be implanted before programming, whereas some centers may program the first side before implanting the second side. This will be something that you should check with your DBS team if you are considering surgery.

PREPARING FOR P-DAY (THE DAY OF PROGRAMMING)

The first thing to realize about the initial programming visit is that it will be long. Remember that each lead in the brain has four contacts near the tip. Stimulation can be delivered through any one of these four contacts. Although the contacts are very close to each other, chances are only one or two of these contacts are at or near the right spot that will help your symptoms. The purpose of the initial programming session is to test all four contacts and find out which one helps your symptoms best. The best contact is the one that helps your symptoms at the lowest setting and gives you side effects only with high settings. (This is somewhat similar to finding a good medication for you—the best one helps your symptoms at the lowest dosage without giving you too many side effects.)

For people living with Parkinson's disease, the initial programming visit is done in the "off" medication state. That means you should not take any of your Parkinson's medications for 12 hours prior to the appointment. Again, this applies only to your Parkinson's medications. You will be allowed to take your other medications as usual. While this will likely make you uncomfortable, it is a necessary part of programming because if you are "on" your medications, your symptoms are likely to be masked, and the clinician who is turning on and adjusting the stimulator will not be able to tell if the stimulation is helping you. DBS centers often make the initial programming session the first appointment of the morning, so that most people do not have to go for too long without their medications. You should bring your Parkinson's medications with you to the appointment, as you will have to take them as soon as the programming visit is over. If you live far away from the clinic that will be doing your initial programming, it may make sense to stay at a nearby hotel the night before the programming for your convenience. People with ET and dystonia typically undergo the procedure only if medications are not helpful, so being "off" medications is not an issue. However, it will still be a fairly long visit.

Someone should accompany you to your initial programming session, as you will not know how your body will respond to the stimulator. It is always helpful to have someone there for support even if things go smoothly. Furthermore, if you are "off" Parkinson's medications, you will be exhausted by the end of the programming session and likely will not be in the mood to drive yourself home.

WHAT HAPPENS ON P-DAY?

Again, it is worth emphasizing that who does your programming is as important as who places the DBS. Many people only research the neurosurgeon, how many individuals he or she has operated on, and what his or her complication rate is. However, once the DBS system is in place, the neurosurgeon is out of the picture (unless there are surgical complications). The person who turns it on and sets the settings will be your friend and contact over the next 3–6 months. This person will work with you to find the settings that benefit you with the least amount of side effects. While the basic principles of programming are rooted in science, programming is also part art. A feel for how someone will tolerate programming is something that is only picked up after much experience.

Who Does the Programming?

The person who turns on your DBS system and finds the best settings is known as the programmer. In most DBS centers, this person is either a neurologist specializing in DBS or a nurse/nurse practitioner working with a neurologist. Occasionally, a neurosurgeon or a nurse working with the neurosurgeon will be the programmer. There is no official certification or minimum amount of training to become a programmer, but by this time, you have probably researched and picked your DBS team because they have a lot of experience with this already.

PROGRAMMING BASICS

Monopolar vs. Bipolar Stimulation

Again, there are four electrodes or contacts at the end of each DBS lead. Depending on the model of the lead placed in your brain, these contacts can be 0.5 or 1 mm apart from each other. If you chose a good neurosurgeon, at least one of those contacts will be in the right spot. Programmers can choose any one of those contacts as the active contact (which means the contact where the stimulation comes out) or cathode (negative electrode). Once the stimulation comes out of the contact, it searches for the anode (positive electrode) to complete an electrical circuit. Thus, the electrical field can be changed to help enhance effect or minimize side effects depending on what the programmer chooses as the cathode and anode.

The most common type of stimulation is called monopolar stimulation. This is where one of the contacts on the lead is the

Monopolar

- One or more contacts active, case positive
- Field diffuses radially
- More clinical effect at lower voltages

Bipolar

- One or more contacts active, neighboring contact positive
- Stimulation field more focused
- Minimizes side effects

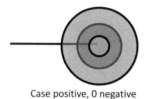

Case positive, 0 negative

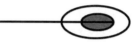

1 positive, 0 negative

Monopolar stimulation vs. bipolar stimulation

active contact or cathode. The battery in your chest serves as the anode. When stimulation comes out of the contact in monopolar stimulation, it spreads out to try and find the anode. If you were to visualize how the electrical stimulation comes out of the contact, picture dropping a pebble in a pond. Where the pebble hits the water would be where the active contact is. The act of dropping this pebble creates waves that go out from the pebble in a radial fashion. This is how stimulation using a monopolar configuration spreads in your brain. Most programmers will start with a monopolar configuration because it is most likely to stimulate the area needed to help your symptoms. However, the downside of monopolar stimulation is that even if it spreads to the correct area, it could spread to an area that you do not want, and thus you would get side effects. In Parkinson's disease, if the lead is placed in the subthalmic nucleus (STN), the nerve fibers that control your face, arms, and legs run right next to the STN. If stimulation spreads beyond the STN and into these nerve fibers, you could get muscle spasms or contractions in these body parts.

If your programmer finds that you get such side effects at low settings, he or she might switch to something called bipolar stimulation. This is where one of the contacts is the cathode or active contact. However, the anode is set at the contact right next to the active contact. This time, when the stimulation comes out of the active contact, it is drawn to the anode right next to it. Thus, the area of stimulation is reduced compared with that of monopolar stimulation, and you are less likely to have side effects. The downside of bipolar stimulation, however, is that you typically have to turn the stimulation to higher settings to get the same response as with monopolar stimulation at lower settings.

Voltage, Frequency, and Pulse Width

In addition to setting which contacts are positive or negative, there are three other variables that your programmer can adjust: voltage, frequency, and pulse width. The electrical stimulation that comes out of the contact can be visualized as a square wave. Each square wave is a pulse of stimulation, and stimulation is delivered constantly to the brain in frequent pulses.

Voltage is measured in volts and refers to how high the pulse gets. Obviously, the higher the voltage, the bigger the pulse. Voltage is the main thing that is adjusted over time because a small increase in voltage tends to give you the most effect on symptoms, whether it is tremor, stiffness, or slowness. Average voltages tend to range from 2 V to 4 V. The higher the voltage is, the more likely the stimulation is to spread to other structures and cause side effects.

Frequency is measured in hertz and refers to how many pulses are given in 1 s. For people with tremor, Parkinson's disease, and dystonia, the frequency typically ranges from 130 to 185 Hz. Frequencies lower than 100 Hz tend not to be as beneficial, although for some people with dystonia, lower frequencies may be helpful.

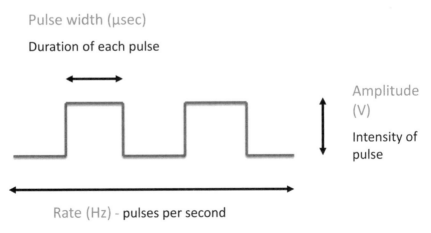

Pulse width (μsec)
Duration of each pulse

Amplitude (V)
Intensity of pulse

Rate (Hz) - pulses per second

Electrical pulse stimulation parameters

There was also a study that suggested that lower frequencies may be more likely to help freezing of gait than higher frequencies in Parkinson's disease.

Pulse width refers to the length of time each pulse lasts. It can be programmed from 60 to 450 μs. For Parkinson's disease and essential tremor, standard pulse widths tend to be between 60 and 120 μs. People with dystonia tend to have much higher pulse widths, with many DBS centers starting at 210 μs. This is because the medical literature has shown that higher pulse widths tend to be more helpful for dystonia symptoms.

Finding the Sweet Spot

On the day of programming, your programmer will do a brief examination to see what your symptoms are. The object of programming is to find the best contact for you, which is the contact that gives you the best effect at the lowest settings. It is important to remember that not all symptoms respond in the same way to DBS. For example, tremor often responds within seconds to a minute after turning on or adjusting stimulation. For those with essential tremor and Parkinson's disease with a noticeable tremor, you will be able to see the stimulator work for you immediately. For the parkinsonian symptoms of bradykinesia (slowness of movement) and rigidity (stiffness), you will have to wait longer before you will notice an improvement. Stiffness improves within minutes, whereas slowness may take minutes to hours before improvement is noticed. People with dystonia have to wait the longest of all. Dystonic symptoms may take weeks to months before getting better after an adjustment.

The stimulator is turned on using a handheld device. This handheld device has a screen that displays which contacts are set as cathodes or anodes, as well as the voltage, pulse width, and frequency. It also gives information as to how long the programmer has been on since the last visit as well as the battery life of your generator. The device uses radio waves to transmit information from the handheld device to the implanted generator in your chest. The radio waves can go through clothing and skin, and so are noninvasive.

Your programmer will turn on stimulation from each of the four contacts on the lead. The pulse width and frequency are typically set at standard parameters, and the voltage is adjusted. With each increase in voltage, you will be expected to report any improvement in symptoms or any side effects. It is important to report everything you feel, even if you do not think it is important. For each contact, your programmer will record the lowest setting where you noticed improvement in symptoms and the lowest setting where you noticed intolerable side effects. Some settings will bring out numbness, tingling, or an electrical shock. Some will bring out muscle spasms. Others will cause slurring of the speech, sweating, anxiety, lightheadedness, or even sadness. However, once the stimulator is programmed, the stimulator is left on, and there should not be any of these side effects. The exception is those individual with essential tremor who may feel a temporary tingling in their hand, arm, or face each time they turn on their stimulator.

After testing each contact, your programmer will select the best contact and put you on your initial settings of voltage, pulse width, and frequency. If you have Parkinson's disease, you may then be asked to take your Parkinson's medications and wait around in the lobby area for a while. Remember that the combination of new stimulation with medications may temporarily increase dyskinesias. Once your medications kick in, if there are too many dyskinesias, your programmer may elect to decrease the amount of stimulation before sending you home. If you have essential tremor or dystonia, you will also be asked to wait around in the lobby area for a while to monitor for side effects. If you do not experience any side effects after an hour or two, you likely will be able to go home.

FUTURE PROGRAMMING VISITS

The initial settings that are programmed at the first visit are rarely ideal. Your programmer will not want to set your stimulator at too high of a setting for fear of causing side effects. The full effects of stimulation sometimes are not seen until the evening or the day after your programming. Programmers who are too aggressive often get phone calls the next day from people because they cannot tolerate the settings. This is somewhat similar to starting medication. Sometimes if you take the highest dose suggested by the pharmacy, you may not be able to tolerate it. But if you start at the smallest possible dose and then increase it slowly over time, you might be able to tolerate your medication better. This "start low and go slow" approach is probably the best way to go about programming.

This means that you will likely have frequent visits over the first few months to have the stimulator adjusted. It is hard to give you an idea of how many programming visits you will need to optimize the settings because it varies widely from person to person. A North American survey of DBS centers reported that in the first month after initial programming, they averaged about 2 programming visits per person with DBS. In months 2–6, there were about 4 visits or 1 per month. In months 6–12, there was an average of 2 programming visits per person or 1 every 3 months. In months 12–24, there was an average of 2 programming visits per person or once every 6 months.

ADJUSTMENT OF MEDICATIONS

Because people with ET and dystonia have failed medications before getting DBS, they usually are not on medications for their condition after surgery. Therefore, this section really is focused toward those living with Parkinson's.

You have to think of DBS as an electrical form of levodopa (the medication typically used for Parkinson's). Levodopa can help tremor, slowness, and stiffness, and so can DBS. However, levodopa can also cause dyskinesias (abnormal involuntary fidgety type movements), and so can DBS. The dyskinesias caused by DBS are usually temporary and last for a few days before the brain adjusts to it.

We have already mentioned that people living with Parkinson's disease can reduce their overall medication dose by about half. However, keep in mind that this is after medications and stimulation settings are optimized. It is unrealistic to think that you can reduce your medications by that much after the first session. More often, you might be able to reduce it only a little bit. Some people may not be able to even tolerate a dose reduction after the first visit. The key here is to remain patient. Some centers will tell you to try and reduce medications after the first programming visit, whereas others will tell you to not change medications. Although there is no standard guide to reducing medications, most people will get there eventually.

Some people may also want to be able to stop their Parkinson's medications entirely. Although that may be possible, it occurs rarely. We like to compare adjusting stimulation and medications to making chili. Think of stimulation as chili powder and the other medications as other spices such as salt and pepper. Very few chilis will taste good with just chili powder alone. Most will need a combination of chili powder, salt, pepper, and other spices. Finding the right combination of spices is what adjusting stimulation and medication is all about. Although it may take some time to find just the right recipe, if you are patient, the end result will be sublime.

NINE

Taking Care of Your DBS System and Other Precautions

Once you have your DBS implanted and programmed, you will be involved in keeping it working properly and preventing it from being damaged or causing harm. There are medical tests and procedures that could turn off your stimulator, cause your stimulator to malfunction, or even lead to stroke or death. Falls or accidents may result in damage to your DBS. We recommend that you and your family or friends become familiar with the precautions that need to be taken to prevent harmful interactions with your DBS.

WHAT IF I FALL OR GET INTO AN ACCIDENT?

While a large component of this chapter will be spent describing the consequences of exposing your DBS to electromagnetic or magnetic fields generated by machines and medical equipment, the most common risk to your DBS is experienced by taking a fall or being involved in an accident. Falling, being involved in a motor vehicle accident, and experiencing some other type of accident are the most frequent causes of device failure. Sudden pulling or jarring that occurs from falling or being involved in an accident can break the small wires in your stimulator lead or extension. The wires can break anywhere along the system, but it usually occurs at one of the connections along the route near the stimulator or the lead. Remember that there are four small wires wrapped within the extension wire that go from the four contacts at the tip of the lead to your stimulator in your chest. It is hoped that, if you experience a break, it will only occur in one of these wires, and the device can be reprogrammed to work around the broken wire using a different wire or contact. Unfortunately, that is not always possible. Broken wires most often require another surgery to fix the DBS.

While you can probably do most of your regular activities after DBS placement, certain activities are just bad ideas. For example, contact sports such as football or rugby should be avoided. Scuba diving may also be dangerous because water pressure could damage the system. When riding in cars, wear your seat belt. If you like to ride bicycles or rollerblade, please wear a helmet to protect your head. The purpose of DBS is to improve your quality of life, and if you find yourself being able to try more activities, we encourage it. However, we would recommend using your common sense to prevent injury.

WHAT ABOUT MAGNETS?

It is possible that your DBS can be turned off by common electromagnetic or magnetic fields. An electromagnetic field is the electric and magnetic force that is detectable around a magnet or an electric current. Electromagnetic or magnetic fields can be generated from a wide variety of sources. Medical equipment, machines, car engines, radios, wireless telephones, handheld power tools, refrigerator doors, and stereo speakers are some of the common sources that can turn off your DBS. Security devices at airports, store entrances, and court buildings could also potentially turn off your device. While your DBS will not be harmed, you may find having your stimulator accidently turned off to be an inconvenience.

You will be given a handheld device when your DBS system is implanted. This handheld device allows you to turn your DBS system on and off, and can also allow you to check whether the system is on or off. Depending on the model of your stimulator, you may also be able to adjust the stimulation settings for your DBS or switch between different settings that the neurologist sets for you. We always suggest that people check every night if their stimulator is on or off before going to bed. The reason for this is that if the stimulator happens to be turned off, you only have to review what happened in the past 24 hours to figure out what could have turned the stimulator off, as the stimulator was on the night before. When you do not check whether the stimulator is on or off each night, and one night you happen to check it because your symptoms are worse, it could have been turned off that day or a couple of days before.

It is also best to use the handheld programmer to check your DBS after having any medical procedure or test or if you have been near a potential electromagnetic field. The airport is a special situation. Remember that going through the metal detectors or even having the wands run over you could potentially turn off the stimulator. When you approach a security entrance at the airport or other secure environment where metal detectors are used, let them know you have a pacemaker and ask to have your security check done by hand. There is no need to say you have DBS or a stimulator because they likely will not know what that is. However, if you use the word "pacemaker," you will be placed in a special line to be hand searched. They may ask you for your ID card that shows you have a pacemaker device, although we have heard from individuals that they rarely have to show it. Some people also carry a letter written by their physicians, just in case.

Whenever you notice your symptoms have suddenly worsened, we recommend that you use your handheld programmer to check your DBS to determine if it was accidentally turned off. See Chapter 10 for instructions on how to do this. You can easily use the programmer to turn it back on.

CAN I GET OTHER MEDICAL PROCEDURES DONE WITH THE DBS SYSTEM?

There are guidelines and certain precautions that need to be applied to those with DBS. The following paragraphs describe the most common guidelines. Further information about the interaction of your DBS with other devices, equipment, or procedures can be provided by the implanting physician or device manufacturer.

Diathermy

The precaution that has the most serious consequences is also the least frequently encountered. People with DBS cannot have diathermy performed anywhere on their body. What is diathermy? Diathermy is a medical treatment that delivers energy and heat within body tissues using high-frequency electrical currents. This energy can be transferred through the DBS system to the brain, causing tissue and nerve damage in the brain, resulting in serious injury or even death. This could happen regardless of where the diathermy treatment is applied on the body. There are *no* circumstances in which diathermy can be performed on an individual with DBS. Diathermy may be called shortwave diathermy, microwave diathermy, therapeutic ultrasound diathermy, and deep heat therapy. It is most commonly used by physical therapists to treat sore achy muscles or by dentists following a painful dental procedure. Diathermy should not be confused with diagnostic ultrasound that is commonly used to obtain images for diagnostic purposes or visualize internal structures in the body.

X-rays or Fluoroscopy

Routine X-rays will not affect your stimulator. However, because you may be exposed to a large electromagnetic field in the X-ray suite, you should check your stimulator to make sure it is still on.

CT and PET (Positron Emission Tomography) Scans

These diagnostic scans will not harm your stimulator and are safe for those with DBS. After the scan, be sure to check your stimulator to make sure it is still on.

Magnetic Resonance Imaging

There is concern for those with DBS when undergoing MRI. Because MRI uses a large magnet and radio waves to create images, MRI is not safe in most circumstances. It can heat the DBS system. This heat may be transmitted through the wires and out the contacts at the tip of the lead, which may burn the surrounding brain tissue. Although it is possible for an individual with DBS to have an MRI, the scan should only be done at a center that is familiar with DBS because there are specific rules that must be followed. First, only a *brain* MRI can be performed with a DBS system in place. This brain MRI can only be performed using a head coil with the MRI strength being 1.5 Tesla or less. The head coil is the part of the machine that actually takes the pictures of the brain. It looks like a basket and slides over the person's head during the MRI scan. To get MRI pictures of other parts of the body, other types of coils are used. An individual with DBS should never have a total body or full body radio frequency coil MRI that extends over the chest. This means that spine, body, shoulder, knee, or other MRIs of the body cannot be done.

Before undergoing a brain MRI, the stimulator should be programmed to 0 V and then turned off. This is because the MRI will switch the DBS system on and off multiple times throughout the entire scan. If your DBS stimulator settings are set at their normal voltage, this frequent on/off toggling could be uncomfortable, causing tingling sensations or temporary shocks. The handheld programmer does not have the capability to turn the stimulator down to 0 V, so someone from the DBS team (or someone familiar with DBS if you are not getting the MRI at your DBS center) will need to turn the stimulator down to 0 V. Although there does not seem to be any problems with MRIs as long as the above guidelines are followed, many academic medical centers have radiology departments that will not perform MRIs in anyone with a DBS system in place, not even brain MRIs.

We recommend that, just in case, MRI be avoided if possible for people with DBS. If you are scheduled to undergo an MRI, you should inform your physician or the MRI department of these precautions.

Electrocautery

Electrocautery is commonly used during surgical procedures. It utilizes an electrical current to stop bleeding vessels or tissues. It should be used with caution in those with DBS. Monopolar or unipolar electrocautery should *not* be used. If electrocautery is necessary, a bipolar device may be used as long as the DBS is set at 0 V and turned off. The difference between monopolar and bipolar electrocautery is somewhat similar to the difference between monopolar and bipolar settings in DBS (reviewed in Chapter 8). In monopolar electrocautery, the electrical current flows from the cautery pen through the subject's body. In bipolar cautery, the electrical current flows only from one tip of the cauterizer to the other, and a limited amount of tissue is affected in between. Because of the difference in the mechanism, the power setting required for bipolar cautery devices is lower than with monopolar electrocautery.

If you have DBS and are undergoing a surgical procedure, your surgeon should be aware that you have a DBS device and that only bipolar electrocautery should be used. Furthermore, the surgeon should know that the ground lead needs to be placed as far away as possible from your DBS such as on the leg.

Cardiac Pacemakers

There is a small risk that the DBS will cross talk or interfere with a cardiac pacemaker. However, if the pacemaker is placed at least 10 inches from the DBS, and there is intraoperative testing to check for interference, those with DBS can safely have a cardiac pacemaker.

Emergency Cardio Pulmonary Resuscitation (CPR)

We are often asked about the precautions that should be used if an individual with DBS suffers a cardiac arrest and needs emergency CPR and defibrillation (electric shock to the heart). Clearly, those who suffer a life-threatening emergency that requires resuscitation should be defibrillated if necessary. However, it is likely that the DBS will be damaged. If possible, place the defibrillator pads at least 2 inches from the stimulator and use the lowest defibrillation settings possible.

Electrocardiogram (EKG) or Electroencephalogram (EEG)

An EKG monitors the electrical activity of your heart and reveals your heart rhythm and heart rate. It is done by applying 12 sticky pads to your chest, arm, and leg. An EEG is similar, except that it monitors the electrical activity of your brain. These tests are safe for those with DBS. However, the DBS is likely to produce interference or artifact that will make it difficult to interpret the EKG or EEG. The DBS can be temporarily turned off with your hand-held programmer while the EKG or EEG is being done. However, if someone requires continuous monitoring, like in an intensive care unit, it may be difficult to leave the DBS off continuously.

Ultrasound

Ultrasound is also called sonography. This is a medical procedure that uses high-frequency sound waves to produce images of organs, tissues, or blood flow inside the body. The sound waves come out of a device called a transducer. Diagnostic ultrasound is safe for those with DBS. To eliminate artifact from the DBS, however, it is recommended that the DBS be set at 0 V and then turned off using the physician programmer. The transducer should be kept at least 6 in. away from the stimulator.

Lithotripsy

Lithotripsy is a treatment that uses shock waves to break up kidney stones. It can damage the DBS system. However, if it is necessary to perform lithotripsy in someone with DBS, then the DBS should be shielded, and the stimulator should be programmed to 0 V and turned off with the physician programmer.

Dental Work

In general, dental procedures are safe for those with implanted DBS systems, except for diathermy (mentioned earlier in this chapter). However, electric dental equipment such as drills or X-ray machines should be kept far away from the DBS generator and wires in the neck and scalp. For extensive dental work, or for suspected tooth abscess (infection), we recommend that those with DBS be treated with antibiotics prior to having the work done.

Radiation Therapy

In the event an individual with DBS needs to undergo radiation therapy to treat cancer, this can be accomplished safely. We recommend that the radiation beams be kept as far away from the DBS system (including stimulator and wires) as much as possible and apply a protective shield over the DBS stimulator.

Mammogram (Breast X-ray)

Mammograms can be performed safely in those with DBS. Care should be taken to avoid compressing the DBS. Make sure you tell the technician about your DBS so that undue pressure is not applied on the DBS or connector.

Industrial Equipment

Industrial plants or environments with large electrical equipment should be avoided as they may affect your DBS. Examples of equipment to avoid include arc welding equipment, power lines, and electric generators.

Household Appliances

Small household appliances and equipment should not affect the DBS. However, if power tools or equipment are held close enough to the DBS generator, they can turn it off. Microwave ovens can be safely used by those with DBS.

Taking care of your DBS is essential to keep it working properly and to prevent it from being damaged or causing harm. Certain medical procedures or tests are contraindicated for those with DBS. However, most medical equipment and procedures are compatible so that your DBS should not interfere with any necessary medical care. DBS failure is more commonly the result of falls or accidents rather than medical equipment or procedures. We recommend that you and your family or friends become familiar with the precautions that were identified in this chapter and refer to this anytime you have questions about the compatibility of your DBS. If more information is needed, or if a procedure is proposed that was not included in this chapter, contact the device manufacturer or the implanting physician before undergoing the procedure.

TEN

Stimulator Battery Maintenance and Checkups

*I*n Chapter 8, we discussed what happens at the initial programming visit. After arriving to the clinic in the morning, the DBS programmer checks all of the contacts at the tip of the DBS lead to find the "sweet spot," the place where stimulation has the best effect on your symptoms with the least amount of side effects. If you have Parkinson's disease, this visit is done "off medications," that is, it is done without taking your Parkinson's medications the night before. If you have essential tremor or dystonia, you may take your medications in the morning. All subsequent programming visits for people living with Parkinson's are usually able to be done in the "on" medication state, although some centers may still occasionally have you come in "off" medications to troubleshoot problems.

In general, you may have several visits over the first 6 months after the initial programming (see Chapter 8) if you have essential tremor or Parkinson's disease. For people with dystonia, it may take weeks for you to notice an improvement with a stimulator change. As a result, dystonia programming visits are spread out more, maybe once every 4 weeks or so. No matter if you have Parkinson's, tremor, or dystonia, once your stimulation parameters have stabilized, the follow-up DBS checkup visits are spread further apart. The DBS checkup visit schedule may end up being once every 3–6 months for people with Parkinson's and once every 6–12 months for people living with essential tremor and dystonia. More frequent checkups may be needed as the battery nears its end of life.

WHAT HAPPENS AT A DBS CHECKUP?

The main purpose of a DBS checkup is to check the stimulator battery. Unfortunately, the existing stimulators on the market do not have a warning beep or warning light to let you know the stimulator battery is failing. However, the DBS neurologist or programmer can quickly check the stimulator and see whether the battery is failing. This is often called "interrogating the stimulator."

When the programmer uses the programming device to interrogate the stimulator, he or she can get a reading on your battery. Depending on the model of your stimulator, the readings are slightly different. With the Soletra model made by Medtronic, Inc., the battery level stays at 3.72 V for most of the life of the battery. When the battery level starts to fall below 3.70 V, then the programmer knows that the battery is approaching end-of-life. At 3.60 V, the level starts to drop rapidly, and by 3.40 V, the battery needs to be replaced immediately. Different centers have different thresholds at which they do battery replacements. If you can be monitored frequently, and if surgical battery replacement can be scheduled within a day or two, then you can wait until the battery drops to 3.40 V. At some centers, it may take a longer time to schedule surgery, so these centers may opt to change the stimulator battery earlier.

With the Kinetra model made by Medtronic, Inc., the stimulator should be monitored more closely when the battery level reaches 2.44 V and should be replaced quickly when it gets to 2.36 V. The Kinetra has an additional feature in that it will tell the programmer that less than 20% of the battery has been used, or it will say that 45%–70% of the battery has been used.

The Activa PC/RC model by Medtronic, Inc., will let the DBS programmer know that the battery still has life by showing "OK" on the physician's programming screen. When the stimulator is running low, "ERI" will appear on the physician's programmer. Once an "ERI" warning appears, there is approximately 3 months before the stimulator battery runs out. It will show "EOL" when the battery life is gone.

A second purpose of the DBS checkup is to make sure that the stimulator is still delivering stimulation to your brain appropriately. The programmer will check your settings to make sure that they are still the same as the end of the previous visit. The programmer can also check if your stimulator has been on the entire time since your last visit or if it has only been on 67% of the time (seen with people with essential tremor because they turn their stimulators off at night). In addition, impedance and amount of current are checked. These are measures of how well the electrical stimulation is being delivered to the brain. The impedance is the resistance of an electric circuit to current and is measured in ohms. If the impedance is high, it could suggest that there is a broken lead or connection problem. If the impedance is really low, it could suggest a short circuit. People can sometimes feel a short circuit if they have consistent electrical shocks along the extension wire or over the stimulator battery.

Finally, the DBS checkup is your chance to tell the DBS programmer or neurologist how you have been doing. If the stimulation settings are not controlling your symptoms quite as well, it may be time to increase them. If you are having side effects, then it may be time to lower the voltage or try a bipolar stimulation configuration to cut down on side effects.

HOW LONG DOES THE STIMULATOR BATTERY LAST?

The battery in the stimulator can last anywhere from 3 to 5 years. This is a wide range, and it is because some people need higher stimulation settings than others. If your symptoms can be controlled with low stimulation settings, the stimulator is likely to last more toward 5 years. If you need higher stimulation settings to control your symptoms, then the stimulator will run out of juice more quickly.

The stimulators of individuals with essential tremor tend to last the longest. This is because, typically, tremor can be controlled at lower stimulation settings. In addition, people living with essential tremor are instructed to turn their stimulators off at night. Why? The main problem in essential tremor is shaking of the hands, which interferes with the ability to use them. As a result, people may be unable to write, eat, or drink from a cup with one hand, etc. When people with essential tremor are sleeping, they do not need to use their hands, so the stimulator can be turned off. They can then turn it back on in the morning when they wake up. This cuts down on the amount of time the stimulator is working, and batteries tend to last more than 5 years.

On the other hand, people with Parkinson's disease will still have symptoms overnight. The slowness and stiffness that occur with Parkinson's may interfere with the ability to get comfortable when trying to fall asleep. These symptoms may also make it difficult to get up in the middle of the night to go to the bathroom. People living with Parkinson's who have rest tremors will often say that the tremor prevents them from falling asleep. As a result, people with Parkinson's are instructed to leave their stimulators on all the time. This allows them to feel more relaxed, and many report better sleep because of the stimulator. Because their stimulators are on all night, the battery generally lasts between 3 and 5 years.

Individuals with dystonia usually need high stimulation settings to help their symptoms. Voltages and pulse widths are typically set higher for dystonia than for essential tremor and Parkinson's disease. As a result, their stimulators tend to last at most 3 years, although there will be exceptions to this rule.

DBS HANDHELD DEVICE

Soletra Handheld Device (Access Review Therapy Controller)

Each stimulator available on the market has its own handheld device. The Soletra stimulator's handheld device is called the Access Review Therapy Controller. This device has four buttons on the front, two gray and two blue. The blue buttons to the right are the on and off buttons. The on button is above, and the off button is below. To turn your stimulator on, you would place the Access Review device over your stimulator and press the on button until you hear a beep. Then look at the back. There are three lights to the left that should be green. If the top one is lit and green, then the stimulator is on. To turn the stimulator off, place the Access Review device over your stimulator and press the off button until you hear a beep. Then look at the back. If there is an amber light that lights up on the right side of the controller, then your stimulator is off.

You can check if the stimulator is on by using the bottom gray button on the left. To do so, place the Access Review device over your stimulator and press the bottom gray button until you hear a beep. Then look at the back. If the topmost green light is lit on the back, then it is on. If the amber light on the right is lit on the back, then it is off.

Kinetra Handheld Device (Access Therapy Controller)

The Kinetra's handheld device is called the Access Therapy Controller. On this device, the on/off buttons are the two blue buttons in the middle, with the top one being on and the bottom one being off. To turn your stimulator on, you would place the Access Therapy Controller over your stimulator and press the on button until you hear a beep. Then look at the back. There are three lights to the left that

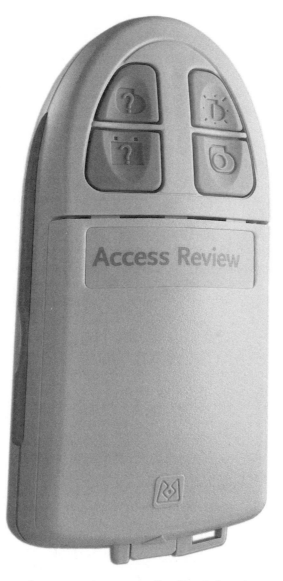

Access review controller (for Soletra)

should be green. If the top one is lit and green, then the stimulator is on. To turn the stimulator off, place the Access Therapy Controller device over your stimulator and press the off button until you hear a beep. Then look at the back. If the amber light on the right is lit, then it is off.

The Access Therapy Controller has four gray buttons with arrows on them. The two buttons on the left are for controlling the

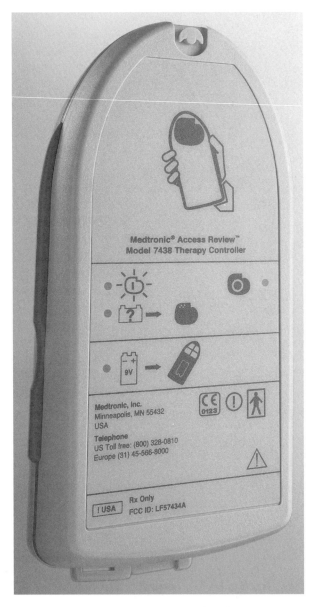

Access devices, back side

right side of the body, whereas the two buttons on the right are for controlling the left side of the body. These buttons can be set by the DBS programmer to allow you to increase your voltage up or down. If the DBS programmer does not enable this function, you can use any of the gray buttons to check if your stimulator is on.

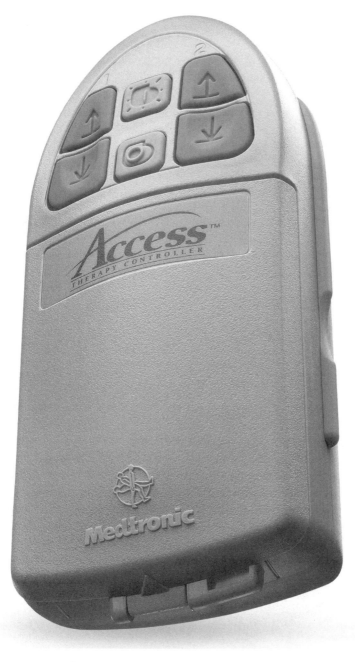

Access therapy controller (for Kinetra)

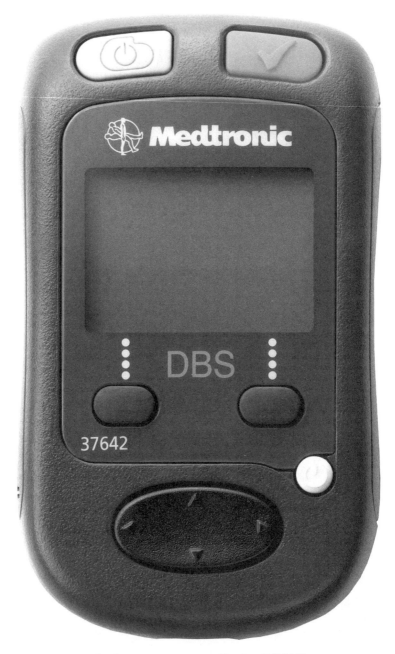

Patient programmer (Activa PC/RC)

Activa PC/RC Handheld Device (Patient Programmer)

The handheld device that comes with the Activa PC or RC stimulators is called the Patient Programmer and looks different from the other handhelds. It has a simple and advanced mode. The simple mode allows you to check the status of your stimulator battery and turn it on or off. The advanced mode can be set by your neurologist and will allow you to change your stimulator settings or toggle between preset settings.

To turn your stimulator off with this device, hold the Patient Programmer over the stimulator while pressing the gray "On/Off" key located at the top left corner of the device. The display screen on the handheld device will say "On" or "Off" depending on whether the stimulator is on or off. You can also use the orange "check" button at the top right of the device to check if your stimulator is on or off. To do this, simply hold the Patient Programmer over the stimulator while pressing the orange "check" button and then looking at the display screen.

Changing your stimulator settings or switching between preset settings is a little more complex. If you and your neurologist decide that having these options would be helpful for you, your neurologist should explain how to switch your stimulator settings using the device.

REPLACING THE STIMULATOR

Replacing the stimulator is a relatively simple operation that is done on an outpatient basis. It is usually performed under general anesthesia so that you are completely comfortable. In the operating room, you will be placed on the operating table, and the skin over the stimulator will be thoroughly cleaned and sterilized. An incision is made at the stimulator site, which is usually in the chest. The original incision site is reopened. After the incision is made, the old stimulator is removed. Once the old stimulator is removed, the new stimulator can be placed in the same skin pocket in the same location under the skin. Care is taken when placing the new stimulator to be sure not to damage the extension lead where it attaches to the stimulator. The incision is usually closed with sutures, but surgical adhesive or staples can also be used.

Because this is a simple outpatient procedure, you can plan on being discharged from the recovery room after you are feeling well. Prior to discharge, the new stimulator will be set back to your old stimulator's settings. Once you are awake, and without nausea or other adverse effects, you will be discharged to home. You will experience some pain and swelling at the incision and stimulator site. Prescriptions for mild pain medication are given upon your discharge. You will also need to have someone drive you home. Upon discharge, you will be given instructions about resuming activity, diet, and medication.

Once you are home, make sure to become familiar with the instructions given to you. You should not drive until your physician gives approval. You should be active, but avoid exaggerated movements such as swinging a golf club or vacuuming.

The risks related to replacing the stimulator are low. The most significant risk is infection. Infection can occur despite administering antibiotics in the operating room. Signs of infection are redness at the stimulator, drainage, increased swelling, and fever. Infections are treated aggressively so that they do not result in having to remove the entire DBS. If you suspect an infection, it is important that you call your surgeon immediately.

Another risk to consider is possible damage to the extension wire where it is connected to the stimulator. As discussed in previous chapters, the extension wire is a tube that encases four tiny wire within. Extreme care must be taken to avoid damaging these tiny wires when disconnecting from the old stimulator and connecting to the new stimulator. If the extension gets damaged, it will need to be replaced surgically.

My Symptoms Are Not Under Control — Troubleshooting Your System

Although we hope everything has gone smoothly with your DBS procedure and programming, nothing ever goes perfectly. In this chapter, we go over cases where the symptoms are not under control. The first few cases go over situations where the symptoms were never helped even with the DBS surgery. The ones after that go over situations where the DBS was working for a while and then suddenly stopped working. We hope these examples help you understand potential problems with the DBS. The first people to ask if things are not going right are your DBS programmer and DBS neurologist. Although many of the examples relate to Parkinson's disease, the same concepts can be applied to people with essential tremor and dystonia as well.

DBS NEVER HELPED SYMPTOMS IN THE FIRST PLACE

Poor DBS Candidate

A 68-year-old man had Parkinson's symptoms for about 6 years prior to DBS surgery. When he first went to a neurologist, he was found to have a "stone face" and tremors of his hands (although they were noticeable only when he used his hands), but his most prominent problem was frequent falling and a shuffling gait with frequent episodes where he felt like he was "stuck in place." His neurologist started carbidopa/ levodopa with entacapone, and there was minimal change in his gait and no decrease in falls. He was tried on many other medications for Parkinson's but had side effects with all of them. He needed to use a walker after 3 years and was wheelchair-bound after 6 years. Increasing the levodopa did not improve his walking ability, but he felt better on the medication. Five years into the course of his disease, he started developing speech problems as well. He was sent to a neurosurgeon who thought this individual might benefit from STN DBS. Unfortunately, he did not improve after turning the stimulators on, despite multiple DBS adjustments over a year.

Unfortunately, this person was not an appropriate DBS candidate in the first place. The first criterion for DBS surgery for someone living with Parkinson's is a diagnosis of Parkinson's without evidence of an atypical parkinsonian syndrome. This person's clinical presentation and progression are atypical of Parkinson's disease. Frequent falls are extremely rare within the first few years of a diagnosis of Parkinson's disease. Although falling and balance problems can occur, they typically happen later in the course of Parkinson's disease. This person also did not have the typical rest tremor that is seen in Parkinson's disease. The second criterion for DBS surgery in an individual with Parkinson's disease is a robust and sustained response to levodopa. This person did not have any clear response to levodopa. Remember, in Parkinson's, DBS does not make you better than the medications. During this person's best "on" time, he still needed a walker, so it was unrealistic to expect that his walking would improve with stimulation. Ultimately, the person found his way to a DBS center, and he was found to have eye movement problems that suggested a diagnosis of progressive supranuclear palsy, which is an atypical parkinsonian syndrome. The eye movement problems may not have been present at the time of surgery, which makes diagnosis of this condition difficult. Nevertheless, there were many other reasons to suspect that DBS would not be appropriate for this individual besides the incorrect diagnosis.

For this reason, we suggest that prior to considering DBS, you should be seen by a movement disorder specialist. Whether you have Parkinson's disease, essential tremor, or dystonia, the movement disorder specialist evaluation is a way to confirm your diagnosis. DBS will not be successful if you have a diagnosis that will not respond to stimulation. Most DBS centers have a movement disorder neurologist who performs all of the screening evaluations. We believe that selection for DBS should involve an experienced multidisciplinary team that performs detailed preoperative assessments. If you are interested in DBS, please read Chapters 3 and 4 to get a better idea of the selection criteria for DBS and how to choose your DBS team. Deciding to undergo DBS is a big step, and you want to make sure that you have the best team in place to insure your success.

Poor Electrode Placement

This 65-year-old man was diagnosed with Parkinson's disease 10 years prior to DBS surgery. He was maintained on carbidopa/levodopa for many years, but 3 years into the course of the disease, he started to experience wearing-off symptoms. Pramipexole and entacapone were added over the next few years and seemed to smooth out his motor function. He then started to develop dyskinesias with his medication regimen. When his medications worked, he was able to perform his daily activities without difficulty. When he wore off, he felt aching in his legs and had a freezing gait. He was deemed an appropriate candidate for DBS and underwent bilateral STN DBS surgery in 2007. A few days after being programmed, he started developing unusual behaviors such as placing a dining room chair on the front seat of the car to go to the grocery or put what was needed in the oven in the freezer and vice versa. These behaviors went away with programming, but this person never felt that the stimulation helped the motor symptoms of his Parkinson's disease. He was programmed for a year before being sent to a specialized DBS center for evaluation. On imaging, one of his electrodes was found to be misplaced. His symptoms improved dramatically after replacing the electrode.

This was an appropriate candidate for DBS. He had a diagnosis of Parkinson's disease with a progression in symptoms that was typical. He had a robust and sustained response to levodopa for many years, but started to have motor fluctuations despite optimal medication management. He also did not seem to have any significant memory problems or depression prior to surgery. However, he never really had a great response to stimulation, and in fact, he started to have unusual effects from the stimulation. In an appropriate candidate, the first step would be to obtain an imaging study of the head to look for a misplaced electrode.

There are two different ways to obtain brain imaging: magnetic resonance imaging (MRI) or computed tomography (CT) (please see Chapter 9 for more details). Please remember that if your physician orders an MRI to look for a misplaced lead, there are certain safety precautions that the MRI technician has to follow. In some centers, the radiology department or center will not perform MRI on anyone with a DBS system, so CTs are ordered. There are pluses and minuses to both techniques.

Sometimes a lead that is suboptimally placed can be overcome by DBS programming. This is why it is important to have not only a good neurosurgeon who can put the lead in the right place but also a good neurologist or nurse programmer who knows how to program the DBS device well. However, if the lead is way off target, replacement has to be considered. A study by two DBS centers has recently found that about half of their "DBS failures" were due to misplaced leads. While having to go through another surgery may seem horrible, at least lead misplacement could potentially be corrected, giving you a good chance at improving your symptoms.

Programming Problem

A 58-year-old man underwent bilateral STN DBS for Parkinson's disease. His main symptom was a severe tremor, but he also had some slowness in movements. After surgery, his neurologist programmed him for 1 year. He had an improvement in his slowness but never noticed a significant improvement in his tremors. Brain imaging revealed that his electrodes were accurately placed. After referral to someone with more experience in programming DBS, he walked out of the office without a trace of tremor.

This person also seems like an appropriate candidate for DBS surgery. He has a diagnosis of Parkinson's disease, but has tremor that is disabling despite being treated with medications. Remember that tremor is the one feature of Parkinson's disease that may not respond to medications but could respond to stimulation. If an individual did not respond to stimulation, but seems like a candidate, the next step would be to check if the stimulators were placed appropriately. In this case, imaging confirmed good placement of the electrodes. After that, reprogramming would be the next step. This person's neurologist had little experience programming stimulators, having only one other individual in his practice with this condition. An initial testing of the leads was never performed, so the optimal contact was not known. Remember that at the end of each lead, there are four different contacts where the stimulation comes out. For most cases, only one or two of these contacts are within the targeted structure (the thalamus, STN, or GPi). Therefore, testing should be done on all of the contacts to see which one helps the symptoms the most. This person was brought in, and each of the contacts on the left and right sides was tested. It was found that by changing to a different contact, the person had significant improvement in his tremors and walked out happy.

This case illustrates the need to have someone experienced with programming the DBS system. We suspect that many individuals may be told that the DBS was a failure, when, in fact, many could be turned into "successes" by referring them to a DBS center for evaluation.

Failure to Achieve Expectations

Case 1. A 73-year-old woman with a 12-year history of Parkinson's disease underwent bilateral STN DBS surgery. Prior to surgery, she was responsive to levodopa, but her levodopa only worked about 50% of the waking day. When she was "off" medication, she needed assistance with all basic activities of daily living, and she could not walk at all. When she was "on" medication, she could dress and bathe independently, although slowly. She could walk in her "on" state but needed the help of a walker in order to walk without falling. Her main problems prior to surgery when "on" medications, however, were severe dyskinesias (involuntary movements) at the peak of her levodopa doses that were sometimes painful. After STN DBS surgery, her dyskinesias improved significantly, and she felt "on" for most of the day. She presented for a second opinion because the DBS was not helping her to walk independently.

Remember that for Parkinson's disease, DBS does not make someone better than their best "on" medication state. This woman could not walk independently prior to surgery even with Parkinson's disease medications. Thus, it is unrealistic to expect to walk independently after DBS surgery. By reducing dyskinesias and improving "off" time, this surgery should be considered a success. However, because it did not meet up her expectations, she thought it was a failure. While it is the job of the DBS team to let you know what the surgery will and will not improve for you specifically, it may not always be communicated to you clearly. We would recommend that you have an honest discussion with your neurologist and neurosurgeon about your own goals and expectations prior to surgery. Write these goals down on a piece of paper and ask your DBS team whether or not they are realistic. Your expectations can make a big difference in how you assess the success of your surgery.

Case 2. A 22-year-old man had generalized dystonia for most of his life. There was no injury at birth, but he developed dystonic postures of his body as he became older. Despite these problems, he was able to work and live independently, although he needed to put in extra effort sometimes in order to accomplish basic tasks that everyone else takes for granted. The most bothersome aspect of his dystonia was that he did not look "normal." Also his speech was not always clear. He underwent GPi DBS with the hope that these symptoms would improve. Prior to surgery, he was counseled that the effect of stimulation likely would not improve his symptoms 100%, espe-cially speech, and he appeared to understand. The DBS surgery improved his dystonia by approximately 50%, and he had a significantly easier time performing manual tasks. However, he was disappointed in the surgery and called his DBS a failure because he could not walk "normally."

Unlike the individual in the first case, this person was counseled about realistic expectations prior to surgery, especially regarding the fact that he likely would still have some dystonia if the surgery was a success. The goal of the surgery according to the DBS team was to improve his symptoms so that he would have an easier time per-forming tasks. By doing so, his quality of life would also improve. They thought that this goal was communicated to him. However, in hindsight, the goal of the surgery in this man's eyes was to make him "normal." Because it did not accomplish that, the surgery was a failure. This case re-emphasizes the fact that you should write out your goals clearly prior to surgery and discuss them with your DBS team. If you have chosen a team that you trust, they should be will-ing to discuss these issues with you.

DBS WORKED AND SUDDENLY STOPPED WORKING

Infection

A 70-year-old man who underwent left Vim DBS for essential tremor had good control of his right-hand tremor after surgery. Approximately 2 months after surgery, he noticed a decrease in his tremor control, as well as scalp tenderness. He reported catching his comb on his surgery scar frequently over the past couple of weeks. Examination of the incision site on top of the head showed redness and swelling, suspicious for an infection. This individual eventually had to have his DBS system taken out and underwent a course of IV antibiotics. After his infection was treated, he opted to have his DBS lead replaced. After replacement, his tremor control was once again good.

Infections may be a complication of any surgery. An infection typically happens within the first few months of DBS placement and is likely due to poor wound care. Dirt or bacteria from hair, dirty hands scratching the incision site, soap, or shampoo could potentially get in a wound before it heals completely and lay the groundwork for an infection. That is why some DBS surgeons pre-fer shaving the entire head, so that there is less of a chance for these things to infect the wound. Others may not shave the head, but will restrict you from using shampoo and combs near the incision site until it is completely healed. In either case, it is important to keep the incision sites clean until they heal up properly. Once there is an infection, it can be difficult to treat. If the infection is small, a course of oral or IV antibiotics may be enough to treat the infection. However, often, the entire system has to be taken out, along with a course of IV antibiotics, before it is safe to put DBS hardware back in. It is important that you follow the directions of the neurosurgeon for the first few months after surgery to prevent infection.

Stimulator Off or at End of Life

Case 1. A 64-year-old man with Parkinson's disease underwent DBS surgery and had marked improvement in symptoms for 6 months, and he was seen urgently because of recurring Parkinson's disease symptoms over a 3-day period. He was given a device that allowed him to check whether his stimulator was on or off at the time of surgery, but did not know where he had placed it. In the clinic, the stimulator was checked, and it was discovered to be off. After turning the stimulator back on, his symptoms improved. The person had used a power saw in his shed a few days ago for the first time after surgery, which turned his stimulator off.

Case 2. A 24-year-old woman with generalized dystonia underwent bilateral GPi surgery 4 years ago with good benefit. She was seen urgently because of worsening dystonic symptoms over a period of 1 week. When the stimulator was checked in clinic, it would not respond to the controller, suggesting that the battery was at end-of-life. The woman's battery was replaced, and she continued to experience a good benefit from stimulation.

Some people, specifically those with tremor, will notice almost immediately when their stimulators are turned off. That is because tremor seems to respond quickly (within minutes and sometimes within seconds) to electrical stimulation. For other symptoms such as bradykinesia and rigidity of Parkinson's, the full effect of a change in stimulation may not be seen for days. With dystonia, the changes may take weeks to be seen. People living with essential tremor are often encouraged to turn their stimulators off at night and on in the morning, so if the tremor does not respond when they try to turn the stimulator on, it is likely at the end-of-life and needs to be changed. For those living with Parkinson's disease, the stimulators are on 24 hours a day. For these people, we recommend that they check to see if their stimulator is on once a day. Nowadays, everyone should be given a device after surgery that allows them to check whether the stimulator is on, as well as allow them to turn the stimulator on or off. That way, if their stimulator is ever turned off for any reason, they can look back on their previous day to figure out what might have turned their stimulator off. Devices that generate strong magnetic fields, such as the refrigerator seal, mouthpiece of a phone, metal detectors, power tools, and even the remote of a Toyota Prius, have been reported to switch the DBS stimulators off. This seems to be less of a problem than several years ago, but if you notice that your symptom control changes suddenly or over a few days, you should first check your stimulator to see if it is on. If it is, you should then contact your DBS team to see if your stimulator battery has run out. Most stimulators can last anywhere from 3 to 5 years.

Other Hardware Malfunction

A 54-year-old woman with essential tremor underwent left Vim DBS and had significant improvement in her right-hand tremor for 2 years. However, she reported that her tremor control deteriorated suddenly 1 week prior to her clinic visit. When the stimulator was checked, it was turned on, and the battery was not close to end-of-life. Checking other stimulation parameters demonstrated a high impedance and low current, suggesting an open circuit. X-rays of the head and neck revealed that the extension wire from the stimulator to the lead was kinked. This person had a lead fracture, and tremor control was regained after replacing the extension.

There are other hardware problems that can result in a relatively rapid loss of symptom control. One such problem is a lead fracture. If your DBS programmer suspects a lead fracture, they will often order an X-ray of the head and chest to identify it. The reasons for a lead fracture are unclear, and although sudden and violent movements potentially could result in lead fractures, they often happen without a past history of trauma or sudden movement. Again, if you experience a sudden loss in symptom control, you should first check to see if your stimulator is still on. If it is, then you should make an appointment with your DBS programmer to check if the battery is still working and to check if you could have a possible lead fracture.

DBS SLOWLY STOPPED WORKING OVER TIME

Lead Migration

This 35-year-old woman underwent bilateral GPi DBS for generalized dystonia. She had a good response after about 6 months of stimulation, with about a 70% reduction in severity. About 9 months after her surgery, she presented for a regular follow-up in the DBS clinic and reported that her dystonia had gradually worsened over the past 2–3 months. She checked her stimulator religiously every day and reported that it had never been turned off. Her stimulation parameters were checked and did not show any abnormalities. Upon reimaging her electrodes, it was found that the right electrode had moved approximately 1 cm from previous imaging studies. Her electrode was repositioned in the proper spot without complications, and she again was able to report a 50% reduction in dystonic symptoms compared with before surgery.

Lead migration is not common, but it certainly does happen. If there is worsening of symptoms, lead migration should be one of the considerations. An imaging study compared with one taken immediately after the surgery should show if the electrode had moved. It is unclear why the leads should move over time, although anchoring devices sometimes have been blamed. These anchoring devices are basically plastic caps that fit in the hole that was drilled in your skull at the time of surgery. They are supposed to keep the lead in place, but sometimes they malfunction or the lead is not secured well before the surgeon closes the scalp. Children who often have DBS placed for dystonia and then grow may also be more likely to have lead migration. In the case described above, the lead had to be repositioned, but in some cases, the stimulator can be reprogrammed successfully by switching to an alternate DBS contact.

Disease Progression

This 73-year-old man with Parkinson's disease has had STN DBS for 5 years. He had good control of tremor after surgery and had an improvement in his medication "on" time after surgery. He was happy with control of his motor symptoms for 4 years after surgery, but at that point, he started to notice problems with his balance. Over the past year, he has progressed from walking independently to needing a walker. He has developed freezing episodes that occur at any time throughout the day and do not correlate with when he needs to take his medications. Increasing his levodopa did not help his freezing, neither did increasing or decreasing his stimulation parameters. Brain imaging showed that the leads were in the right place and had not migrated.

Sometimes when a symptom is not optimally controlled, it may be due to progression or worsening of the Parkinson's disease, essential tremor, or dystonia, even in cases with an optimally placed electrode that has been working well for a long period of time. Of course, all effort should be made to identify a correctable cause for inadequate symptom control, such as the stimulator being turned off, battery end-of-life, lead fracture, and lead migration. After that, the stimulators should be adjusted to see if the individual simply needs more stimulation. However, if increasing stimulation does not help, progression of disease is certainly a high possibility. *Remember that DBS is not a cure.* In this case, it has been well established that freezing and other symptoms that do not respond well to levodopa also do not respond well to stimulation, with the exception of tremor.

Tolerance/Habituation

This 58-year-old woman with essential tremor had excellent control of her hand tremor for 5 years after DBS surgery. After that, her tremor control seemed to decline. Now 7 years after surgery, she still has an improvement in tremor when she turns her stimulator on, but it is still noticeable. For the first 5 years after surgery, the tremor used to disappear with the stimulator turned on. Imaging has shown that the lead has not migrated and is optimally placed. Increasing the stimulator over the years improved the tremor minimally, and now will cause sustained tingling of the right side of the face and arm if turned up any higher. Multiple trials of DBS adjustments, including trying other contacts and parameters, failed to improve the tremor further.

DBS tolerance seems to happen to individuals with essential tremor, but not dystonia or Parkinson's disease. In such cases, tremor is controlled over a long period of time (more than 1 year, but often for many years), and then this benefit is lost. It cannot be explained by lead migration or other hardware malfunction or improper programming. It also cannot be explained by disease progression because the loss of symptom control occurs over a relatively short period of time. It is unknown why tolerance occurs. When this happens, some DBS centers may offer an ablative procedure such as a thalamotomy. This involves lesioning the thalamus (i.e., killing the cells) and can be effective for tremor, although it is an irreversible procedure.

TWELVE

Health Risks and Possible Complications in Surgery

THINKING ABOUT THE RISKS OF SURGERY

In any type of therapy, whether surgical or medical, one of the most important considerations is that of the risks compared to the benefits for that particular individual. Each of us is unique, with our own risk and benefit characteristics. Some of us are very sensitive to medications, whereas others tolerate them well. Some experience a rapid progression of disease symptoms over time, whereas others experience a slow and more stable course. Some of us have other medical conditions that complicate therapy, whereas others suffer from one condition and nothing else.

In addition to our risk–benefit characteristics, each of us has our own risk tolerance. For example, although you may be willing to take an experimental medication if there is even a small chance that it will improve our quality of life, others may only wish to take medications that have a well-established track record. Some of us may look forward to surgery as a quick way to make progress in our care; others may wish to avoid surgery at all costs.

Since each of us differs in our risk characteristics and risk tolerance, it is all the more important that we clearly understand the risks involved with a major surgery like DBS. In this chapter, we will examine the risks of DBS that are to be weighed against the potential benefits that were discussed in Chapter 2.

RISKS OF DBS SURGERY AND WHAT IS DONE TO MINIMIZE THEM

Choosing to pursue DBS therapy involves an evaluation process as well as a two-stage surgery. Each of these steps has some risk associated with them. These risks may range from the relatively minor, like feeling anxious during an MRI scan, to the most major, like having an infection or a stroke. In the following sections, we describe each of the common risks associated with the evaluation process and the surgery, as well as some uncommon ones, and what the DBS team does to minimize these risks to individuals.

Claustrophobia

Claustrophobia is the fear of enclosed spaces. Some of us feel anxious or even panicky when we are in a small space such as an elevator, a crowded room, or an MRI scanner. In preparation for DBS surgery, everyone will get pictures taken of their brain with an MRI in order for the neurosurgeon and neurologist to be sure that there are no structural problems with the brain that would interfere with the effectiveness of the surgery. In addition, most people will have MRI imaging just prior to surgery to allow the neurosurgeon to accurately place the DBS lead. The MRI uses strong magnetic fields to get a clear picture of the brain. The most accurate and highest resolution MRI scans are performed with the individual lying in a narrow tube. You may have heard of something called an "open" MRI. This type of MRI is less claustrophobic because the individual is placed in a wider tube. However, to make the "open" MRI less claustrophobic, the quality of the picture is sacrificed. Because being able to see the borders of the brain target is important to make sure the lead is placed optimally, DBS targeting really cannot be performed on an "open" MRI. Although mirrors are often positioned to allow the person to look beyond the tube, the process of having an MRI scan can trigger discomfort in people who are susceptible to claustrophobia. During the first of these MRI scans, these people may be given a mild sedative to help with the anxiety. This can also be done on the day of surgery, although these sedatives have the potential to interfere with the surgery itself and should be discussed with the neurosurgeon. In very extreme circumstances, the MRI scans may be performed with the individual under anesthesia and fully asleep.

Discomfort and Fatigue

During the DBS evaluation and surgery, there may be several portions that can be fatiguing or uncomfortable. For each of us, our tolerance for fatigue and discomfort differs. One of the major goals of the DBS team is to ensure that these unpleasant experiences are minimized, allowing for the best possible outcome. Minor discomfort and fatigue is experienced most often during the neuropsychological evaluation, where people complete numerous tests of thinking and memory over a couple of hours. Although not necessarily uncomfortable, thinking hard can make people feel drained. Think back to your days in school and how you felt after a big test. You may have been excited when it was over but, at the same time, may have felt tired.

People living with Parkinson's will have to undergo an off/on evaluation, where they are evaluated after not having taken their medications overnight. Because Parkinson's medications help tremor, slowness, and stiffness, being off medications for such a long period of time may be exhausting. Therefore, any testing done during the off-medication state may have potential to cause fatigue. By allowing people to have breaks during any testing, the DBS team tries to minimize fatigue.

The surgery itself can also be quite tiring and potentially uncomfortable. During the first stage of surgery, in which the leads are positioned within the brain and secured to the skull, the individual is awake and may be required to sit in a single position for up to several hours. To reduce discomfort and fatigue, the operating table on which the person is positioned is usually padded well. In addition, some centers may provide earphones and music to listen to during the surgery. Finally, a member of the DBS team may be present in the operating room to attend to any needs the person may have as they arise during surgery and to help keep the team aware of any discomfort that the individual may be experiencing or questions that come to mind.

DBS surgery is stressful and may produce anxiety. For those who already have an anxiety disorder, the problem can become worse during surgery. For those who experience anxiety that cannot be adequately controlled during surgery, it is possible that surgery may have to be stopped.

Pain during the surgery itself is also a common concern. To minimize pain, the neurosurgeon numbs the scalp in any location where the person may experience pain. The numbing medication that is used is chosen to last for the duration of the surgery. When the numbing effect has reached the desired level, people may remain aware of what the neurosurgeon is doing, but usually feel no more than the mildest sensations.

After the surgery, the individual can also expect to have some pain or discomfort. Interestingly enough, the brain itself has no sensory fibers and does not feel pain. However, just like any other cut in the skin, the surgical incision sites may be uncomfortable or even painful while healing, and the skin in the region of the incisions may feel abnormal for a number of weeks. The placement of wires underneath the skin also can cause soreness. The soreness may last for 2–3 weeks after surgery. Approximately one in six people will report headaches for a few weeks after DBS surgery. To reduce discomfort due to surgical pain, the DBS team usually prescribes oral pain medication that can be taken for a few weeks after each DBS surgery.

Problems of Lead Location

Just like real estate value, the effectiveness of DBS surgery is about "location, location, location." Whether for Parkinson's disease, ET, or dystonia, the optimal location for the DBS lead in the brain is a target area about the size of a small pea and is located close to the center of the skull. Much of the technology associated with DBS surgery focuses on ensuring the most accurate lead placement possible, as described in detail in Chapter 7. Depending on the technique, the neurosurgeon may use MRI scans, frame-based targeting, microelectrode recording, and intraoperative X-rays to make sure that the lead is placed precisely at its intended location. However, the most important check of lead location during the DBS surgery is neurological testing in the operating room to look for motor, sensory, and other side effects. In many institutions, a movement disorder neurologist performs this testing before the neurosurgeon locks the DBS lead into its permanent location.

Motor Side Effects   Motor side effects are those that affect movement. Each of the three most common targets of DBS is located in close proximity to nerve fibers that control movement. For the STN, the target for many individuals with Parkinson's disease, fibers controlling movement of the hand, face, and eyes are quite close to the optimal target location. The target for essential tremor, the VIM nucleus of the thalamus, is just toward the center of the brain from the fibers controlling movement, and the target GPi for Parkinson's disease and dystonia is just to the outside of these same fibers.

To make sure that the lead is not located too close to these motor nerve fibers, the neurologist or the neurosurgeon will examine the movement of an individual's eyes, face, and limbs while temporarily turning on the DBS system in the operating room. When eye movements are affected, people may comment that they see double when the system is turned on. When nerve fibers controlling the face and limbs are affected, people may feel a clenching of their fingers or toes or a pulling sensation in the face due to contracting muscles. When such motor side effects are encountered, the neurosurgeon will typically relocate the electrode to a location further away from the motor fibers for that target.

Sensory Side Effects   The targets of DBS are also close to nerve fibers carrying sensory information from the spinal cord to the brain. One of the important relay stations for signals coming from the body is the thalamus, and the DBS target for tremor, the VIM nucleus of the thalamus, is located just in front of this region. The STN sits just below the thalamus (hence the term subthalamic), in front of some of the sensory fibers coming from the spinal cord to the thalamus. Finally, the GPi, a DBS target for Parkinson's disease and dystonia, is just above and to the side of fibers carrying signals from the eye to the rest of the brain. As a result of turning the DBS system on and testing for effects during the surgery, many people report tingling sensations in their face, arm, or legs, and in the case of GPi stimulation, may experience flashes of light. If the stimulation is troublesome to the individual at the stimulation levels needed to help control the person's symptoms, the neurosurgeon and neurologist may decide to move the electrode to a new location a few millimeters away.

Voice Side Effects   In addition to effects on movement and on sensation, DBS can affect speech. For many people living with Parkinson's disease, the voice becoming quieter over time is a major communication issue. For people living with essential tremor and dystonia, the shaky or strained voice that can sometimes be heard also affects communication and may cause some to be socially embarrassed. Particularly for the VIM and STN targets, DBS can affect the voice. This is most significant in the VIM nucleus of the thalamus, especially when DBS leads are being placed on both the left and right sides. DBS leads placed into the GPi typically do not affect the voice, except through motor-fiber effects on the muscles of the face and the throat. In some centers, a speech pathologist, a member of the team with specialized training to examine the voice, may be available to examine the individual in the operating room. Examination by a speech pathologist allows voice changes to be determined with maximal sensitivity, allowing the DBS lead to be repositioned if necessary.

Confusion

The brain and spinal cord are normally bathed in a special waterlike solution called cerebrospinal fluid (CSF). During DBS surgery, after the coverings of the brain are opened, CSF may be replaced partially by air. The presence of air in the skull can produce temporary confusion, which may be described by some as "cloudiness," "fogginess," or "fuzzy-headedness." In addition, the insertion of the DBS electrode can result in a small amount of swelling along the path in which the electrode travels. This swelling, called edema, is temporary and can also produce confusion. In essentially all cases, confusion due to the replacement of CSF by air or due to temporary swelling in the brain improves by itself over a few days. To reduce confusion, the neurosurgeon typically takes steps during surgery to minimize the escape of CSF through the opened coverings of the brain.

Another reason for confusion following DBS surgery in people living with Parkinson's disease results from being off Parkinson's medications on the day of surgery. Some people are able to tolerate the off-medication state very well, whereas others become temporarily confused. Whether due to the surgical or medical effects of the procedure, up to one in twenty people (5%) may experience some temporary confusion after DBS surgery. Confusion following DBS surgery may result in hospitalization for 1 to 2 days longer after the surgery.

Seizure

Seizures are bursts of electrical activity in the brain that are not well controlled. Such bursts of electrical activity can result in abnormal movements, changes in thinking, or even unconsciousness. Any operation on the brain or any process that irritates the surface of the brain, such as DBS, can produce a seizure. In addition, seizures may be due to bleeding within or on the surface of the brain, an infection or inflammation in the brain, or changes in the chemical balance of the blood or CSF. About one in one hundred people having a DBS operation may have a seizure. To prevent seizures, neurosurgeons give people antiseizure medications beforehand, if their expectation of a seizure is high enough. Under routine circumstances, antiseizure medications are only given if there is some evidence of a change in the brain that is likely to result in a seizure. Rates of seizures for DBS surgery are no higher than other similar brain surgeries and lower than more invasive surgeries such as brain-tumor operations. Repeated seizures after DBS surgery are very rare.

Stroke

A stroke is a change in the functioning of the brain that lasts for over 24 hours. There are two types of strokes. The first one is called ischemic stroke. Ischemic strokes occur because of the interruption of blood supply to a region of the brain. When the blood does not get to a part of the brain, it does not receive oxygen and can die. The second type of stroke is called hemorrhagic. This happens when a blood vessel in the brain ruptures and blood pours into a region of the brain. This pushes on surrounding brain tissue, causing damage.

Ischemic strokes during DBS surgery are very rare. Fewer than one in one hundred people may experience such strokes associated with DBS surgery. The risk of bleeding with insertion of the electrode into the brain and causing a hemorrhagic stroke is higher. Around one in one hundred people undergoing a DBS operation will experience a hemorrhage.

Circulation Problems

During a DBS operation, individuals may experience changes in their heart and blood pressure. Since the placement of the DBS leads is performed with the individual awake, certain people faint during the procedure. Rates of fainting during DBS operations are around one in thirty individuals.

The DBS procedure may be long, and the person undergoing the procedure does not get an opportunity to move around a lot. This puts individuals getting the procedure at a higher risk of a deep vein thrombosis or a blood clot in the legs. The dangerous part about having a deep vein thrombosis in the legs is that it could travel to the lungs and cause a pulmonary embolism. Pulmonary embolisms occur when the blood supply to the lung is blocked and can result in shortness of breath. These are rare and may need to be treated with strong blood thinners for a few months after surgery.

In addition, people may rarely experience changes in their heart rhythm or may even have a heart attack during DBS surgery. To keep the risks of circulation problems as low as possible, all individuals being evaluated for DBS that are suspected of heart disease are usually evaluated and cleared by a cardiologist, in addition to the usual evaluation by an anesthesiologist.

Infection

Infection is one of the greatest concerns following any DBS operation. The ability of the body to fight infection around any artificial device or material inside the body is reduced compared to normal. As a result, approximately one in twenty-five DBS people may experience an infection.

A change in the skin color (redness) overlying the stimulator, along the extension, or around incision sites suggests infection. If you see this, you should contact your DBS team immediately. In minor cases, the infection may involve the skin only and can be treated effectively with antibiotics taken by mouth. Fever and drainage of fluid from the incision sites would suggest a more severe infection of the DBS system. In such cases, IV antibiotics may be utilized. Finally, when an infection is able to surround a portion of the DBS device, the DBS system may have to be partially or completely removed to allow the immune system to rid the body of infection. This is usually seen with a CT or MRI scan. When a DBS system has to be taken out due to infection, an individual is typically placed on antibiotics for several weeks. This does not mean that a person cannot get the DBS system placed again. Many may be able to undergo replacement of the DBS system a few months later after discussion with the DBS team.

BALANCING THE RISKS AND BENEFITS

Each of us uses a unique and individual approach to think about risk based on our experiences. Some of us are more comfortable with risk, whereas others are less so. It is particularly difficult to weigh the risks associated with rare but very serious complications, of the sort that can occur with DBS surgery. The tendency is to look to our medical providers and to ask, "What would you do?" However, what we would do may be different from what you would do. Therefore, we recommend that you ask enough questions to understand the risks and the benefits of DBS surgery. We individualize the risk assessment through a comprehensive preoperative evaluation. We are certainly willing to share our views of whether, given an individual's level of risk, we would consider having the surgery ourselves. However, ultimately, we believe that it is important that everyone makes an individual choice together with their friends, family, and other loved ones.

Complications for DBS are close to that of any brain surgery and may include:

- Bleeding in the brain
- Stroke
- Infection
- Confusion
- Seizure
- Speech problems
- Breathing problems
- Heart and other circulation problems

One rule of thumb that is helpful to many when making these decisions is that, with DBS surgery, there is a nineteen in twenty chance that the surgery will go without complication and that they will be very happy with the result. That leaves a one in twenty chance that an individual will have a negative outcome. It is this one in twenty chance of negative outcome that must be weighed by each person against the impact that their Parkinson's disease, tremor, or dystonia is having upon their lives. In our experience, people may take a year or more before committing to DBS surgery. This is because undergoing DBS surgery is a big decision and should not be made on a whim. If you would rather live with the disability that your symptoms cause rather than taking this one in twenty chance of a bad outcome, then DBS surgery is not for you. However, if this risk is low enough given the potential benefits that you might gain, then you owe it to yourself to look into the surgery a little bit more.

THIRTEEN

Long-Term Clinical and Side Effects

*I*n the last chapter, we talked about some of the risks of the DBS surgery itself, as well as some of the side effects that occur when the stimulator is first turned on. In this chapter, we will talk about some of the effects of DBS that have been reported long term.

LONG-TERM CLINICAL EFFECTS OF DBS

Parkinson's Disease

The question that most people ask is how long the effects of DBS last. For Parkinson's disease, we now have data that show that DBS can control the main motor symptoms of Parkinson's disease, namely, tremor, slowness, and stiffness, for at least 10 years. However, because DBS was developed in the late 1980s, there are individuals who have had their DBS systems for even longer. Each DBS center probably has a handful of people who have had their DBS systems in for a long time and are still doing relatively well. This does not mean that DBS is a cure for Parkinson's disease. In fact, many things tend to worsen over time in people with Parkinson's who have undergone DBS. Speech and balance problems have been reported in most of the long-term studies of DBS for Parkinson's disease. While speech problems certainly may be due to the stimulation and will be mentioned as a long-term side effect of DBS later in this chapter, part of the speech problems are due to progression of the disease. The balance problems that occur over time in people with Parkinson's disease are also thought to be due to disease progression. Over time, individuals may develop what is called postural instability. This refers to a person's inability to keep standing if something knocks them off balance. This is an unfortunate problem of advanced Parkinson's disease that does not respond to stimulation or medication. Nevertheless, tremor, stiffness, and slowness are still improved 10 years after surgery in Parkinson's disease, so the effects are pretty long lasting.

Essential Tremor

For essential tremor, the effect on tremor is also long term, with evidence that tremor can be improved by up to 90% and maintained for at least 7 years or more. However, some centers have reported that the effect of DBS does seem to decrease over time. There is also the issue of tolerance (discussed in Chapter 11), where the tremor control from stimulation is lost over time and seems to happen only in people with essential tremor. The reason for this is unknown.

Dystonia

There have been reports of individuals benefitting from DBS for generalized dystonia for up to 10 years. These are people with a genetic form of dystonia, called DYT1 dystonia. There are also people with other forms of dystonia, such as cervical dystonia, whose improvement has been maintained for up to 3 years.

LONG-TERM SIDE EFFECTS OF DBS

It should be mentioned that there seem to be relatively little long-term side effects in people with dystonia who undergo DBS. The main ones appear to be possible lead migration or wire fractures, which are mostly seen in children with dystonia who outgrow their leads. There also seem to be relatively little long-term side effects to thalamic stimulation for essential tremor. Most of the long-term side effects listed below are seen in people with Parkinson's who undergo DBS, although when they occur in essential tremor or dystonia, they will be mentioned as well.

Speech

Speech can definitely be affected by DBS. Problems with speech are most commonly seen after DBS surgery for essential tremor, where leads are placed in the VIM nucleus of the thalamus, and Parkinson's disease, where leads are placed in the subthalamic nucleus.

The nerve fibers that control the muscles responsible for speech are very close to the thalamus. As discussed in the last chapter, if the DBS lead is placed slightly lateral within the VIM nucleus, it is more likely to cause speech problems. Remember that if the stimulation is set at a monopolar setting, the stimulation spreads out from the lead in a radial fashion. The higher the voltage setting is, the more it is likely to spread. If someone needs a high setting to control his or her tremor, speech may be affected. Although this can occur when it is placed only on one side, the likelihood of problems increases when leads are placed on both sides. This is why most centers typically place a unilateral lead for essential tremor. When the stimulation spreads to the motor fibers controlling speech, the speech can sound strained, or it can sound slurred, as when people are drunk. Sometimes the DBS programmer can reduce the effect on speech by changing the stimulation to a bipolar setting, which concentrates the stimulation around the contact, but sometimes tremor cannot be completely controlled this way. It may be a choice between good tremor control with some speech problems or sub-optimal tremor control with less effect on speech in these particular cases.

For Parkinson's individuals undergoing STN DBS surgery, the stimulation can certainly spread to speech fibers, although the problems are less prominent than with VIM stimulation in essential tremor. The problem with Parkinson's disease is that speech normally worsens slowly as time goes on. Therefore, it can sometimes be unclear if speech issues are due to stimulation or to disease progression. Sometimes it is due to both. If it is due to stimulation, the speech can sound strained or strangled, or sometimes slurred. When the speech over time gets soft, raspy, or low, then it is usually attributed to disease progression. Either way, problems with speech can lead to communication issues and are very frustrating to both that person and their family.

Speech problems sometimes can be helped by speech therapy. Speech therapy teaches you techniques to help you speak louder and enunciate more clearly. There are different types of philosophies regarding speech therapy out there. One of the most popular regimens is the Lee Silverman Voice Therapy (LSVT), which focuses on thinking and speaking loudly.

Balance

Balance problems are typically seen in people with Parkinson's disease after DBS, but may also be seen in people with essential tremor after DBS as well. Most of the time, balance problems are seen within the first 6 months after surgery in individuals with Parkinson's, as the stimulation is being increased and the medications are being decreased. This happens because your body is trying to get used to all of the changes. The balance problems are typically gone once the stimulation and medications are optimized. A small proportion of people with Parkinson's disease will continue to have balance problems, however. This may be due to a number of reasons. Some people continue to get dyskinesias despite the DBS (see next section for more details). These dyskinesias can throw you off balance. Sometimes the stimulation has spread to the nerve fibers controlling the muscles in your legs. When this happens, you may not have full control of your leg, and it may involuntarily turn in or move out. Sometimes it may be because the medications were reduced too quickly. In any of these cases, you should bring these problems up with your DBS neurologist and work with him or her to improve the problem. Sometimes physical therapy may also help you to regain your balance.

The balance problems seen in people with essential tremor are usually due to a lightheadedness that is experienced when the stimulators are turned up. This lightheadedness feeling seems to be more noticeable when DBS leads are placed on both sides of the brain. This is another reason why DBS centers may tend to recommend DBS leads on only one side for essential tremor. However, balance problems have also been reported in people with essential tremor who have not undergone DBS. In fact, there have been reports that the cerebellum is also affected in essential tremor. The cerebellum is the part of the brain that coordinates movement. When the cerebellum does not work correctly, people may walk or reach for things like they are drunk. In essential tremor, these balance problems are usually not quite that severe, but physical therapy seems to be helpful.

Dyskinesias

This is a problem seen only with Parkinson's disease and can occur either with STN or GPi stimulation. Dyskinesias are a long-term side effect from chronic use of levodopa. They are involuntary movements of any part of the body that typically increase at the peak of the levodopa dose. Remember that stimulation is like an electrical form of levodopa. Thus, when stimulation is turned on, dyskinesias can be increased. Individuals generally notice a worsening of dyskinesias when the stimulation is turned on or when the stimulation settings are turned up. However, this usually lasts a couple of days at most and then wanes as the brain becomes used to the stimulation. Sometimes Parkinson's disease medications are also reduced, which can also improve dyskinesias.

Although dyskinesias are typically reduced over the long term with DBS surgery, there are some people in whom we are unable to reduce dyskinesias. These individuals are very sensitive to the stimulation, and even small increases in stimulation result in dyskinesias that, unfortunately, do not diminish after a few days. With these people, trying to find the right combination of medication and stimulation can be very difficult. One approach is to try and increase the stimulation slowly, over a period of a year, rather than the usual 3–6 months. Another approach is to send the stimulation through one of the higher contacts, which may suppress dyskinesias.

Weight Gain

This problem seems to be a concern only for individuals with Parkinson's disease, especially after STN DBS surgery. Weight gain does not seem to be a significant problem for people undergoing DBS surgery for essential tremor or dystonia.

Parkinson's disease itself has been associated with weight loss. In fact, many people living with Parkinson's disease tend to lose weight as the disease progresses. However, after DBS surgery, weight gains of 10%–25% have been reported. There are several theories out there as to why this happens. Many people living with Parkinson's disease undergo DBS because of severe, disabling tremor or significant dyskinesias (abnormal involuntary movements). Because of these movements, such people are in constant motion and thus are burning calories. With DBS controlling the tremor and reducing dyskinesias, these people burn less calories and thus gain weight. Although this theory makes a lot of sense, individuals with Parkinson's who do not have severe dyskinesias or tremor may also gain weight after DBS. We really do not know why this is. It is possible that we are changing some of the circuits in the brain that control our metabolism. Whatever the reason, weight gain is something that can be seen and should be monitored.

We typically encourage everyone undergoing DBS to exercise, which may keep weight gain to a minimum. Exercise is good for general health, an optimistic outlook, and increased energy. There is also evidence that exercise helps with thinking and memory. If you gain weight despite the exercise, we often refer people to a dietician or nutritionist for tips on healthy eating.

Apraxia of Eyelid Opening

Apraxia of eyelid opening is an inability to open the eyes voluntarily. In this condition, the eyes can close by themselves, but people then have difficulty opening them. Many have described having to use their fingers to pry their eyes open. This can be disabling. If you cannot open your eyes quickly, many activities, especially driving, are compromised. Apraxia of eyelid opening seems to occur only in people with Parkinson's undergoing DBS and also seems to be associated with subthalamic nucleus (STN) DBS as opposed to GPi DBS. It can occur in between 2% and 30% of these individuals after STN DBS.

Treatment of apraxia of eyelid opening is with botulinum toxin, commonly known as Botox. Botulinum toxin is injected directly into the eyelids and the muscles around the eyes. It works by blocking the signal from the nerve to the muscle. If the muscle never gets the signal to contract, the muscle relaxes and the eyes open much more easily. In severe cases, when botulinum toxin does not work, individuals can undergo an operation called a frontalis suspension. In this operation, the eyebrow area is connected with the upper eyelid by sutures, located deeply under the skin and not visible to others. This allows a person to use the eyebrows to help open the eyes and can be helpful.

Depression

Depression is something that has been reported to occur after DBS surgery for Parkinson's disease, especially with the STN target. Although rare, it is something that you and your DBS team should monitor. In some cases, the depression can be so severe that some individuals have tried to commit suicide. Virtually every DBS center, if it operates on enough people, will have one or two of these cases. Originally, it was thought to occur because the expectations of the individual were not met. However, there have been reports of people who have been satisfied with the results of their DBS but, despite that, tried to commit suicide. There was a report in the *New England Journal of Medicine* of a woman who started to become tearful when the DBS was turned on and did not feel that way when the DBS was turned off. The sadness that engulfed this person only happened when the lowest contacts of the DBS lead were stimulated. It turned out that the lowest contacts were probably outside and below the STN. Providing stimulation to this area was thought to stimulate fibers that were responsible for mood. This was evidence that depression could be "hard-wired" in the brain and that stimulation could activate these moods. Other studies have shown that people with a history of severe depression, especially those needing hospitalization for their depression, seem to be at highest risk for developing depression after DBS surgery. This is why DBS centers try to screen people for the presence of depression before operating. Although we still do not have a great handle on who will develop depression after surgery, it certainly makes sense not to operate on someone who is in the throes of depression.

Some people will experience worsening depression after DBS, and this may be related to the site of the electrodes. You should have any depressive or other psychiatric symptoms (anxiety, apathy, psychosis, or impulsivity) evaluated before surgery to be as safe as possible.

Cognition

Cognition, or your ability to think and remember things, is something that can definitely change after DBS surgery. Again, this does not seem to be much of a problem in people with essential tremor or dystonia, as long-term cognitive studies in these people do not show much change in formal neuropsychological testing.

In Parkinson's disease, however, changes in cognition have been clearly reported. This seems to be reported more often in people with their leads placed in the STN than in those with their leads placed in the GPi. The most common change that we see after surgery is a decline in verbal fluency. Verbal fluency is a test where you are asked to name as many words beginning with the letter "F" as you can in 1 min. There are many variations on this task, with some asking you to name as many animals or vegetables in a minute and others using different letters. This task tests the organization of your brain and the ability of your brain to remember what you have said while trying to come up with new ones. After DBS surgery, the number of words that a person can produce in 1 min declines. This is the most consistent finding regarding cognition in the medical literature on DBS. However, it is still unclear what a decline in verbal fluency means, as many people have declines in this task after DBS but do not complain of problems in daily life. Others may complain of memory problems and may have changes in memory tasks on formal testing, but their performance on verbal fluency may not change. Overall, long-term studies in people living with Parkinson's disease undergoing DBS have shown that mild cognitive decline is fairly common. However, all centers clearly have some people who have more than mild changes in thinking and memory after surgery.

A reason why cognition changes after DBS is that by placing hardware through the brain, you are disrupting the connections from one part of the brain to another. It is also possible that stimulation itself is affecting your thought processes, although it has been difficult to separate whether changes in cognition are due to the surgery itself or due to stimulation. One thing that is clear is that certain individuals worsen cognitively after surgery. People who already have significant problems with their thinking and memory are more likely to experience problems after surgery. This is why neuropsychological testing is done before the surgery. Those who are on the borderline of dementia or who have dementia could likely worsen after the surgery. With DBS surgery, we are trying to improve your quality of life. If we worsen your cognition to the point that dementia is an issue, then we are not improving quality of life.

Sometimes when cognition worsens after surgery, it can also be due to progression of Parkinson's disease. It is estimated that up to half of the people living with Parkinson's may develop dementia. There are medications that can be given to help such individuals. These medications are called cholinesterase inhibitors, and they increase the amount of acetylcholine, a chemical in the brain. The cholinesterase inhibitors were initially developed for the treatment of Alzheimer's disease, although they have certainly proven to be helpful for cognitive problems in Parkinson's as well. The common ones used are donepezil (Aricept) and rivastigmine (Exelon). Only rivastigmine is FDA approved for Parkinson's dementia; however, there are data to suggest that donepezil could be helpful as well. Many clinicians may actually start with donepezil because it is available as a generic medication and is less expensive than rivastigmine. However, rivastigmine is available in a patch form, which may be easier to administer and is definitely better for people with swallowing difficulty.

FOURTEEN

Frequently Asked Questions

DOES INSURANCE COVER THE COST OF THE PROCEDURE?

DBS is FDA-approved and covered by most health insurance companies. Some insurance companies require prior authorization before having surgery, and some do not fully understand DBS and may initially deny coverage. However, usually with some detailed explanation, the decision is reversed. Sometimes insurance denial is based on the false assumption that DBS is experimental. If your diagnosis is Parkinson's disease, tremor, or dystonia, the proposed DBS surgery is approved by the FDA and is *not* experimental. If the DBS surgery is recommended for a different diagnosis, it may indeed be considered experimental and is at risk for denial of coverage. Experimental DBS surgery will require authorization/approval from your insurance company.

DOES THE DBS PROCEDURE NEED TO BE DONE WITH MRI? I HAVE A PACEMAKER AND CANNOT GET AN MRI

The MRI provides the clearest and most detailed pictures of the brain. This is the preferred method to make sure the best outcomes are achieved from surgery. However, DBS surgery can be performed using CT guidance. CT, or computed tomography, is a way of imaging the brain, but the detail in the pictures is not as good as with MRI. This may lead to suboptimal outcomes. CT-guided DBS is easier with VIM nucleus placement (done for essential tremor), as the VIM nucleus is a bigger structure and not as deep. CT-guided DBS is much more technically difficult if the neurosurgeon is trying to place a lead in the STN. Not every neurosurgeon is willing to do DBS surgery with CT guidance, so you should check with the DBS center to make sure they will do CT-guided DBS before making an appointment.

WHERE WOULD YOU PUT THE DBS STIMULATOR IF I ALREADY HAVE A PACEMAKER?

Pacemakers are typically placed in the same pocket in the chest where DBS stimulators are placed. Because pacemakers are placed on the left side of the chest, the DBS stimulator could be placed on the right side of the chest. Another alternative would be to place the DBS stimulator just under the skin in the abdomen. The extension wires from the leads to the stimulator would be longer, which would put it at higher risk for lead fracture, but there is generally more "padding" in the abdomen, so the stimulator does not stick out as much.

WHAT IF THE STIMULATOR BATTERY RUNS OUT? WHAT WILL HAPPEN?

It depends on what your symptoms are. If you have essential tremor, your tremors will not be controlled. While this is an annoyance, it is generally not considered an emergency, but you should contact the DBS team to have the stimulator replaced as soon as possible. If you have Parkinson's disease, the symptoms of tremor, slowness, and stiffness may come back in full force over a couple of days. In some cases, this can be an emergency because you may be unable to move. Remember that you are on less Parkinson's medications now, so the amount you are taking is unlikely to help as much as prior to surgery. If the stimulator battery runs out if you have Parkinson's, you should contact your neurosurgeon or the DBS team as soon as possible. They may tell you to go into the emergency room, and an urgent battery replacement will be scheduled. If you have dystonia, the symptoms of your dystonia may come back over days to weeks. Again, this will be more of an urgent issue, and you should contact the DBS neurosurgeon or DBS team as soon as possible.

WILL OTHERS BE ABLE TO SEE MY DBS STIMULATOR?

Once you are healed, there is very little evidence that can be seen. At some centers, a small amount of hair is shaved above your forehead on the top of your head at the time of Stage I. Most women and some men are able to style their hair in such a way that this is not very noticeable. However, if you have short hair, or no hair, the incisions are likely to be visible to others until you are healed. If your DBS center shaves the entire head, then the incisions will certainly be visible until they heal and your hair grows back. There will be a 2- to 4-inch. incision in the scalp on the top of the head and a smaller incision behind the ear. Once healed, the incisions will leave scars that will be visible on balding heads but are well-covered when hair grows back.

The scalp will have bumps where the holes were drilled. The holes are filled with plastic caps that sit just under the scalp, leaving a small raised area. Again, in those with hair, this is not visible. In balding men, the raised areas on the scalp are more visible.

The extension wire that runs from the lead(s) in the brain to the stimulator is tunneled in the fatty tissue just under the skin. For most, the track of the extension wire is not visible. However, for those that are thin, it may appear as a large vein would, just under the skin.

The stimulator lies under the skin, just below the collar bone. Once healed, there will be a 3- to 5-inch. scar from the incision. The stimulator site will be slightly raised. This is more noticeable in those that are thin. It may be noticeable if one is wearing a bathing suit or low cut blouse. However, this generally is not seen through clothing.

WHY WOULD YOU CHOOSE THE STN AS A SITE FOR PARKINSON'S DISEASE? IT SEEMS THAT IT IS ASSOCIATED WITH MORE PROBLEMS THAN GPI

Most centers implant leads in the STN for Parkinson's disease. This is mostly due to training and comfort with the procedure. In a recent large DBS trial comparing STN to GPi DBS for Parkinson's disease, there was not much difference in the effect on motor symptoms. STN had a slight advantage in that people were able to reduce their medications more. In other studies, GPi is reported to have less depression and fewer problems with cognition after surgery, but in this large DBS trial, there really were not any clinically significant differences in outcome with respect to depression or cognition.

I LIVE ALONE. CAN I HAVE DBS?

It depends on whether you have family or friends that are available to stay with you for a few days after surgery and help you with transportation back and forth for your appointments as well as to and from the hospital. We have found that unless you have someone helping you, the outcome from your DBS will be disappointing. However, if you have willing family and friends who are interested in helping you, as long as you have not suffered any adverse events from surgery, once you have recovered from your DBS, you should be able to return to living alone.

I NEED TREMOR CONTROL IN BOTH OF MY HANDS TO PERFORM MY JOB. CAN I HAVE DBS FOR BOTH HANDS?

If you have Parkinson's disease, you are likely to have bilateral surgery with placement of leads in the STN or GPi and experience tremor control in both hands. If you have essential tremor, lead placement occurs in the VIM nucleus of the thalamus, but often only on one side. This is done to see if there is enough benefit with tremor control in one hand. By doing so, the risk is cut in half. It has been our experience that most people can perform most of their activities with tremor control in one hand. However, if you find that you need both hands to be controlled, it is possible to place a DBS system for the other hand. However, keep in mind that those with bilateral VIM leads for essential tremor often describe problems with speech and balance.

HOW DO I KNOW WHEN TO USE MY DBS?

Individuals with Parkinson's disease or dystonia will be instructed to leave the stimulator on continuously. There is no need to turn off the stimulators, unless undergoing a medical procedure. Those with essential tremor who have leads placed in the VIM can turn the stimulator on or off as needed, depending on when tremor control is needed. Many people turn the stimulator on in the morning upon waking and off at bedtime.

CAN I DO MY OWN PROGRAMMING?

Finding the correct contact on your DBS lead can only be done by the DBS neurologist or nurse who does the initial programming. However, with some of the newer stimulators on the market, they could set it so that you could turn your stimulator voltage up or down within certain limits. The Activa PC made by Medtronic, Inc., also allows the DBS neurologist to set different programs, which would allow you to switch your settings to the exact same settings it was on at the previous visit.

I HAVE ESSENTIAL TREMOR THAT AFFECTS MY VOICE. WILL DBS HELP THE TREMOR IN MY VOICE?

Although DBS is excellent for helping the tremor that is experienced in the hands and arms due to essential tremor, it is unlikely that DBS will help your voice with just a unilateral lead. Although there may be patients who notice a slight improvement in voice with unilateral stimulation, most notice no improvement. With bilateral stimulation, the voice tremor may improve, but bilateral stimulation will often cause slurred speech as well. Botulinum toxin injections are generally more effective for voice tremor than DBS.

WHAT IF SOMETHING LIKE STEM CELLS IS FOUND TO CURE PARKINSON'S DISEASE IN THE NEXT FEW YEARS? DOES UNDERGOING DBS NOW PREVENT ME FROM GETTING THAT TREATMENT?

One of the advantages of DBS is that it is reversible. The stimulation can be turned off, and the hardware can even be taken out. Having

DBS now should not prevent you from getting another treatment in the future if it turns out to be better. However, new treatments such as stem cell therapy will need to be tested in clinical trials before they are approved for use in humans. During the clinical testing phase, you may not be able to participate because clinical trials are often restrictive in their inclusion criteria and will not include people who have had DBS.

Glossary of Terms

apraxia of eyelid opening—A medical condition where people have an inability to open the eyes voluntarily.

atypical parkinsonism—A group of neurological disorders that mimic Parkinson's disease but do not respond to Parkinson's medications.

basal ganglia—A structure within the brain that processes information responsible for initiating and guiding movement. Part of the extrapyramidal system.

bilateral stimulation—When a DBS system is placed only on both sides of the brain.

bipolar stimulation—A way of setting the stimulator so that one of the contacts on the lead is the active (or negative) contact, and the contact next to it is the positive contact. This decreases the amount of spread of electrical current and decreases side effects.

bradykinesia—A slowing of movement. This is the defining feature of Parkinson's disease.

brainstem—The area of the central nervous system that connects the brain to the spinal cord. It is composed of the midbrain, pons, and medulla.

cerebellum—A brain structure that is responsible for coordinating movement.

cerebral cortex—The outermost layer of the brain containing nerve cells that are responsible for brain function.

computed tomography (CT)—A radiological procedure that uses X-rays and a computer to construct a series of pictures of tissues and organs of the body.

contracture—A permanent shortening of muscle, tendon, or scar tissue that produces a deformity, especially around a joint.

deep brain stimulator (DBS)—A device similar to a pacemaker for the heart that sends electrical signals to the brain and can improve the symptoms experienced by people with numerous neurological and psychiatric disorders.

diathermy—A medical treatment that delivers energy and heat within body tissues using high-frequency electric currents.

dopamine—A chemical in the brain that is lost over time in Parkinson's disease.

dyskinesias—Abnormal, involuntary movements of the body caused by Parkinson's medication or DBS.

dystonia—A neurological disorder characterized by sustained contractions of muscles that cause twisting and other abnormal postures. This condition may affect any part of the body and can be generalized. Dystonias can also be primary, which means that they are either genetic or do not have another identifiable cause, or secondary, which means that they are due to something else, like a structural lesion in the brain.

electrocardiogram (EKG)—A recording of the electrical activity of the heart.

electrocautery—This is where an electrical current is used to stop bleeding vessels or tissues.

electroencephalogram (EEG)—A recording of the electrical activity of the brain.

essential tremor—A neurological disorder characterized by tremors of the hands, head, and voice. The tremors are worse when the hands are used and can cause significant embarrassment and disability.

extension—A wire that carries the electrical stimulation from the stimulator to the DBS lead.

extrapyramidal system—One of the motor systems of the brain that help shape and coordinate movement. This brain circuit breaks down our complex movements into sequences of simple ones.

Family Medical Leave Act—A federal law provides employees with up to 12 weeks of unpaid, job-protected leave per year.

frequency—One of the types of stimulation settings. The frequency refers to how many electrical pulses are delivered per second. Typical frequency settings for DBS are 130–185 Hz.

globus pallidus interna (GPi)—Part of the basal ganglia; this is one of the structures targeted for DBS. Placing a lead in this structure can help Parkinson's disease and dystonia.

implantable pulse generator (IPG)—Also known as the stimulator or battery; it is a pacemaker-like device containing a battery that is the source of the electrical signals that eventually travel to the contacts in the DBS lead.

impulse control disorders—These are usually seen with Parkinson's disease treatment. Some people develop strong urges that cannot be controlled. Common examples include pathologic gambling, hypersexuality, or compulsive shopping.

lead—The DBS lead is the portion of the DBS system that is located in the brain.

lead migration—A shifting of the DBS lead over time so that it is no longer where it was originally placed.

magnetic resonance imaging (MRI)—A method that uses magnetic fields to take clear and detailed pictures of the brain.

microelectrode recording—A technology that allows the neurosurgeon, often working with a neurologist or neurophysiologist, to measure the activity of brain cells during DBS surgery.

microlesioning effect—When individuals get a temporary improvement in their symptoms after DBS surgery, usually due to swelling in the brain.

monopolar stimulation—A way of setting the stimulator so that one of the contacts on the lead is the active (or negative) contact with the stimulator being the positive contact. This allows the electrical signals to spread out from the contact in a radial fashion.

motor fluctuations—A phenomenon seen in Parkinson's disease where people go from feeling stiff and slow to normal, to moving excessively, with dyskinesias.

movement disorders—Neurological diseases that affect the ability to produce and control movements of the body.

movement disorder specialist—A neurologist who specializes in the care of people living with movement disorders such as Parkinson's disease, essential tremor, or dystonia.

neurophysiologist—A person who specializes in the interpretation and recording of the electrical activity of the brain during DBS surgery.

neuropsychological examination (or neuropsychological evaluation)—A battery of tests that examine an individual's cognitive (thinking and memory) function. This is usually done prior to DBS surgery and may take a few hours to complete.

neuropsychologist—A licensed psychologist who has completed postdoctoral training in the specialty of neuropsychology and has extensive knowledge of brain structures and brain function.

pallidotomy—A surgical procedure where the nerve cells in the globus pallidus are removed. This was used to help Parkinson's disease.

Parkinson's disease—A neurological disorder characterized by tremors that occur at rest, slowness of movements, and stiffness of the limbs and body. The symptoms are due to a loss of the dopamine-making cells in the brain.

primary motor cortex—The part of the cerebral cortex where all the nerve cells reside that carry signals to the voluntary muscles of the body, such as the face and limbs.

pulse width—This term refers to how wide each electrical pulse is. Typical pulse width settings for DBS are 60–90 µs.

pyramidal system—One of the motor systems of the brain; it is composed of cells that directly control the motor neurons (or nerve cells) of the spinal cord.

rigidity—Stiffness. One of the major symptoms of Parkinson's disease.

speech-language pathologist—Someone who specializes in problems that affect communication.

stereotactic surgery—A form of surgery that makes use of a three-dimensional coordinate system to locate small targets inside the brain.

stimulator—A pacemaker-like device containing a battery that is the source of the electrical signals that eventually travel to the contacts in the DBS lead.

substantia nigra—A small region of the brain located in the midbrain that contains dopamine nerve cells. Loss of these cells is what causes Parkinson's disease.

subthalamic nucleus (STN)—Part of the basal ganglia, the STN is one of the sites for DBS. Targeting this structure helps Parkinson's disease.

tardive dystonia—A secondary dystonia that occurs after long-term exposure to antipsychotic agents or antinausea agents.

thalamotomy—A surgical procedure where the cells in the thalamus are removed. This procedure was often used to help tremor.

thalamus—One of the relay structures of the brain. All of the sensory input from the body goes through here.

tremor—A shaking of a part of a body that is rhythmic.

ultrasound—A medical procedure that uses high-frequency sound waves to produce images of organs, tissues, or blood flow inside the body.

Unified Parkinson Disease Rating Scale (UPDRS)—A commonly used rating scale that rates the severity of Parkinson's symptoms.

unilateral stimulation—When a DBS system is placed only on one side of the brain.

ventralis intermedius (VIM) nucleus—One of the parts of the thalamus; this is where DBS leads are placed for tremor.

voltage—A measure of how strong an electrical pulse is. Typical voltage settings for DBS range from 1 to 4 V.

wearing off—The feeling people living with Parkinson's get at the end of a medication cycle, typically slowness and stiffness.

Support Organizations

GENERAL MOVEMENT DISORDERS

WE MOVE – Worldwide Education and Awareness for Movement Disorders WE MOVE is a not-for-profit organization dedicated to educating and informing patients, professionals, and the public about the latest clinical advances, management, and treatment options for neurologic movement disorders.

WE MOVE
5731 Mosholu Avenue
Bronx, NY 10471
E-mail: wemove@wemove.org
http://www.wemove.org

FOR DEEP BRAIN STIMULATION

DBS-STN.org A website focused on improving quality of life in the DBS-STN community.

DBS-STN.org
The Parkinson Alliance
Post Office Box 308
Kingston, NJ 08528-0308
Phone: 1-800-579-8440
http://www.dbs-stn.org

FOR PARKINSON'S DISEASE

American Parkinson Disease Association A grassroots organization dedicated to easing the burden and finding a cure for Parkinson's disease.

National Office
135 Parkinson Avenue
Staten Island, NY 10305
Phone: 1-800-223-2732 or 718-981-8001
Fax: 718-981-4399
E-mail: apda@apdaparkinson.org
http://www.apdaparkinson.org

The Michael J. Fox Foundation The Michael J. Fox Foundation is dedicated to finding a cure for Parkinson's disease through an aggressively funded research agenda and to ensuring the development of improved therapies for those living with Parkinson's today.

The Michael J. Fox Foundation for Parkinson's Research
Church Street Station
P.O. Box 780
New York, NY 10008-0780
Contact: 1-800-708-7644
E-mail: info@michaeljfox.org
http://www.michaeljfox.org

National Parkinson Foundation The National Parkinson Foundation works every day to improve the quality of Parkinson's care through research, education, and outreach.

National Parkinson Foundation, Inc.
1501 N.W. 9th Avenue/Bob Hope Road
Miami, FL 33136-1494
Toll-free Helpline: 1-800-4PD-INFO (473-4636)
National Headquarters: 1-800-327-4545
E-mail: contact@parkinson.org
http://www.parkinson.org

Parkinson's Disease Foundation (PDF)   The PDF works by funding promising scientific research to find the causes of and a cure for Parkinson's while supporting people with Parkinson's, their families, and caregivers through educational programs and support services.

Main Office
1359 Broadway, Suite 1509
New York, NY 10018
Phone: 212-923-4700
Toll-free Helpline: 800-457-6676
E-mail: info@pdf.org
http://www.pdf.org

FOR ESSENTIAL TREMOR

International Essential Tremor Foundation (IETF)   A nonprofit organization dedicated to providing global educational information, services, and support to those affected by essential tremor, and to health care providers, while promoting and funding essential tremor research.

IETF
PO Box 14005
Lenexa, KS 66285-4005
Toll-free Phone: 888-387-3667
E-mail: info@essentialtremor.org
http://www.essentialtremor.org/Contact-Us

Tremor Action Network   A volunteer nonprofit organization founded by people diagnosed with essential tremor, cervical dystonia (spasmodic torticollis), and tremor-related neurological movement disorders to spread awareness of essential tremor and tremor-related neurological movement disorders by advocating for a cure through research.

Tremor Action Network
P.O. Box 5013
Pleasanton, CA 94566
Phone: 510-681-6565
http://www.tremoraction.org

FOR DYSTONIA

Benign Essential Blepharospasm Research Foundation   A nonprofit foundation whose purpose is to undertake, promote, develop, and carry on the search for the cause and a cure for benign essential blepharospasm and other related disorders and infirmities of the facial musculature.

> Benign Essential Blepharospasm Research Foundation
> P.O. Box 12468
> Beaumont, TX   77726-2468
> Tel: 409-832-0788
> E-mail: bebrf@blepharospasm.org
> http://www.blepharospasm.org/bebrf.html

Dystonia Medical Research Foundation (DMRF)   The DMRF is a non-profit organization dedicated to serving all people with dystonia and their families.

> Dystonia Medical Research Foundation
> One East Wacker Drive, Suite 2810
> Chicago, IL 60601-1905
> Phone: 312-755-0198
> Toll free: 800-377-DYST (3978)
> Fax: 312-803-0138
> E-mail: dystonia@dystonia-foundation.org
> http://www.dystonia-foundation.org

National Spasmodic Torticollis Association   The mission of the National Spasmodic Torticollis Association is to support the needs and well being of affected individuals and families; to promote awareness and education; and to advance research for more treatments and ultimately a cure.

> NSTA Hotline: 1-800-487-8385
> E-mail: NSTAmail@aol.com
> http://www.torticollis.org/contact-nsta.html

ST/Dystonia   ST/Dystonia is a nonprofit organization dedicated to helping people with spasmodic torticollis (ST) or cervical dystonia.

ST/Dystonia
P.O. Box 28
Mukwonago, WI 53149
Phone: 262-560-9534
Toll-free: 888-445-4588
Fax: 262-560-9535
http://www.spasmodictorticollis.org

List of Commonly Prescribed Medications

PARKINSON'S DISEASE

Levodopa Preparations

Carbidopa/levodopa (Sinemet, Sinemet CR, Parcopa)
Carbidopa/levodopa/enatacapone (Stalevo)

Levodopa is the mainstay of Parkinson's disease treatment. It gets changed by the brain's own cells into dopamine, which is deficient in people living with Parkinson's. Levodopa is often combined with carbidopa in the USA or benserazide in other parts of the world. Carbidopa and benserazide prevent breakdown of levodopa in the gut and allow more levodopa to get in the brain. Most people will eventually end up on some form of levodopa. It comes in a regular release form, a long-acting formulation, as well as a formulation that melts in the mouth (Parcopa). There is also a formulation called Stalevo, where levodopa is combined with a COMT inhibitor (see COMT inhibitors below). Common side effects include nausea/vomiting, low blood pressure, lightheadedness with standing, confusion, and dyskinesias.

Dopamine Agonists

Ropinirole (Requip)
Pramipexole (Mirapex)
Rotigotine (Neupro)
Apomorphine (Apokyn)
Cabergoline and Lisuride (available in other countries but not approved for use in the US)

The dopamine agonists are chemically similar to dopamine itself and act on the dopamine receptors of the brain. They help all the motor symptoms of Parkinson's disease, although not quite as effectively as levodopa. Ropinirole and pramipexole are oral forms of the medication. Rotigotine is administered by a patch form. Apomorphine is given through an injection and is very short acting. Common side effects include nausea, lightheadedness with standing, leg swelling sleepiness, hallucinations, and impulse control disorders such as pathologic gambling, hypersexuality, and compulsive shopping.

COMT Inhibitors

Entacapone (Comtan)
Tolcapone (Tasmar)

COMT is an enzyme that breaks down dopamine in the brain. These medications block this enzyme so that dopamine stays around for a longer period of time. These medications are approved for use with levodopa when people develop wearing off. Entacapone is most commonly used and comes in a preparation where it is combined with carbidopa and levodopa (Stalevo). Tolcapone is rarely used because it can cause significant liver problems. The main side effects include discolored urine, dyskinesias, nausea, and diarrhea.

MAO-B Inhibitors

Selegiline (Eldepryl, Deprenyl)
Zydis selegiline (Zelapar)
Rasagiline (Azilect)

Monoamine oxidase (MAO) is another enzyme that breaks down dopamine in the brain, and these medications block it. These medications are approved for early treatment of Parkinson's disease as well as for wearing off and motor fluctuations. They have been suggested to possibly slow down clinical progression, but this has never been proven. Selegiline is broken down into an amphetamine by the body and can cause insomnia. The Zydis selegiline formulation dissolves in the mouth. Common side effects include agitation, insomnia, vivid dreams, and hallucinations. It may also worsen dyskinesias. There is a concern with this class of medications in terms of interactions with tyramine, a chemical that is present in red wine and cheeses. MAO inhibitors also may have a lot of drug–drug interactions with antidepressants, anesthetics, and pain medications.

Amantadine

(Symmetrel)

Amantadine is often used in early Parkinson's for tremor and mild symptoms. It is used in advanced Parkinson's disease to reduce dyskinesias. The common side effects include nausea, confusion, and leg discoloration. It can also contribute to hallucinations.

Anticholinergics

Trihexyphenidyl (Artane)
Benztropine (Cogentin)
Ethopropazine (Parsitan)

These medications are helpful only for tremor in Parkinson's disease, not slowness or stiffness. Their use is limited because of the side effects, which include confusion and other memory issues, hallucinations, drowsiness, dry mouth, dry eyes and blurry vision, and retention of urine.

ESSENTIAL TREMOR

Propranolol

(Inderal)

Propranolol is a beta-blocker, which is a class of medications commonly used to treat high blood pressure, but it is approved by the FDA for essential tremor. The main side effects are a slow heart rate and low blood pressure. Other beta-blockers may be used (atenolol, metoprolol, and nadolol), but they typically are not as good as propranolol.

Primidone

(Mysoline)

This is an antiseizure medicine that is primarily used nowadays to control the tremor seen in essential tremor. Primidone and propranolol are considered the top two medications for essential tremor. Common side effects include sleepiness, balance problems, dizziness, and fatigue.

Benzodiazepines

Clonazepam (Klonopin)
Diazepam (Valium)
Lorazepam (Ativan)
Alprazolam (Xanax)

Although used primarily for anxiety, they can be helpful for tremor as well. Main side effects are sleepiness and dizziness. Some may also experience confusion and problems with thinking and memory. There is a chance of developing addiction or dependence with these medications.

Topiramate

(Topamax)

Topiramate is another antiseizure medication that can control tremor. It is typically used only when a person cannot tolerate or does not respond to propranolol or primidone. Side effects include numbness or tingling, weight loss, fogginess with thinking, or memory loss.

Gabapentin

(Neurontin)

Gabapentin is an antiseizure medication that is also prescribed often for chronic pain. Like topiramate, it can help tremor, but is considered only when individuals fail propranolol or primidone. It is generally well tolerated but can cause sleepiness, fatigue, balance problems, and nausea.

DYSTONIA

Anticholinergics

Trihexyphenidyl (Artane)
Benztropine (Cogentin)
Ethopropazine (Parsitan)

These medications block a chemical in the brain called acetylcholine. It is unclear how these medications help dystonia, but they certainly can. Side effects are common and include confusion and other memory issues, drowsiness, hallucinations, dry mouth, dry eyes and blurry vision, and retention of urine, although young people with dystonia can tolerate high doses without significant side effects.

Benzodiazepines

Clonazepam (Klonopin)
Diazepam (Valium)
Lorazepam (Ativan)
Alprazolam (Xanax)

These medications are also listed under ET but can also help relax spasms in people with dystonia. The common side effects are sleepiness, dizziness, confusion, and problems with thinking and memory. Similar to anticholinergics, some people with dystonia can tolerate high doses of benzodiazepines without significant side effects.

Baclofen

(Lioresal)

Baclofen is a medication that is similar to gamma-aminobutyric acid (GABA), a natural chemical in the body, and is commonly used to treat spasticity and dystonia. It may be taken by mouth or given intrathecally, where it is infused directly into the fluid surrounding the spinal cord. The main side effects include confusion, dizziness or lightheadedness, drowsiness, nausea, and muscle weakness.

Levodopa Preparations

Carbidopa/levodopa (Sinemet, Sinemet CR, Parcopa)
Carbidopa/levodopa/enatacapone (Stalevo)

See this section under Parkinson's disease for how it works and common side effects. There is a small group of dystonia people that respond to levodopa. Although levodopa does not help everyone with dystonia, the ones who respond to it observe a very significant beneficial effect. As a result, most people should at least try this medication before considering DBS surgery or other surgical treatments.

Tetrabenazine

(Xenazine)

Tetrabenazine is a drug that depletes dopamine in the brain. Not everyone with dystonia will respond, but it may be helpful for a select group of individuals. It is available in the USA through a specialty pharmacy. Side effects include depression and parkinsonism.

Botulinum Toxin

onabotulinumtoxinA (Botox)
abobotulinumtoxinA (Dysport)
incobotulinumtoxinA (Xeomin)
rimabotulinumtoxinB (Myobloc)

Botulinum toxin is an injectable medication that blocks the signal from the nerve to the muscle. When the muscle does not get a signal to contract, it relaxes and helps dystonia. Botulinum toxin is considered first-line therapy for dystonias located to one body region. Side effects include bleeding, bruising, pain with injection, and weakness of the muscles injected. Some people can get a flu-like reaction. Botulinum toxin can also spread to other structures throughout the body, such as the diaphragm, and can cause breathing difficulties.

INDEX